Reawakened

Existing Isn't Enough—It's Time to Live!

D0632152

ISBN 978-1-63525-549-2 (Paperback)
ISBN 978-1-63525-550-8 (Digital)

Christian Faith Publishing, Inc.
296 Chestnut Street
Meadville, PA 16335
www.christianfaithpublishing.com

Cover Photo by Bob Capazzo
Graphic Design by Robyn Braik
Surya Namaskar Sun A & Sun B by Angela Derosa
Collaborative Direction and Editing by Lisa Montgomery

Printed in the United States of America

Praise for *Reawakened*

Tina Bilotta's journey from crisis to wholeness is a powerful inspiration for anyone facing challenges here on earth. *Reawakened* is an engaging, accessible, real-world guide on how to get your mojo back, step into your power, and soar!

Tina shares her amazing story of healing, relentlessly getting back up after getting knocked down by heartache, diagnosis, and devastation. With each step, we are encouraged, educated, and inspired to not merely survive but to embrace our own innate ability to heal ourselves… and magnificently thrive.

—davidji, author of *destressifying*

Tina Bilotta continues to set goals for herself and is beyond willing to put in the work to achieve them. On multiple occasions, Tina has proven that no matter what challenges you are faced with, it is in you to surpass all challenges and come out stronger than ever before. With each battle Tina faced, she saw victory in the end because she was adamant to reclaim her wellness. I applaud Tina's authenticity and candid voice throughout her experiences.

Tina's choices are holistic and are based on working naturally through her challenges in order to grow both her mind and body in a healthy, organic way. By all accounts, Tina is deserving of the ultimate breakthrough she has come to. This book is a good read for anyone. It underscores the power we have as human beings to rise above and become the best version of ourselves. In the second half of the book, Tina goes on to share great tips for other individuals to get started with healthy new routines and pays homage to the fact that no two people are alike; everyone needs their own customized health and wellness routine that works for them to achieve their best self.

—Joel Harper, NYC Celebrity Trainer

Understanding the relationship between mind and body has been one of our greatest challenges, and the quest to master it remains even more elusive. The devastation of brain injury can destroy this connection in an instant, and for millions of stroke survivors, they struggle daily in the hopes of regaining just a normal state of being.

Great things can also happen in a moment, like the unexpected phone call I received in my office at NYU Medical Center over six years ago from a young woman who had lost her mother due to a fatal brain hemorrhage.

The conversation was not just about donation money or putting a sign on a hospital wall. It was about a woman who wanted to make a real difference and help others without asking for anything in return. I had never spoken to Tina Bilotta before, but in a true New York minute, Fitness by the Beach and a great friendship were about to begin.

Reawakened reminds us that every day is about new opportunity to celebrate life and help improve ourselves in our desire to be the best we can be both physically and spiritually. Tina Bilotta's journey will give you the tools you need to help yourself and also inspire those around you to do the same. Let today be *your* first day on your personal journey to understand and master your own mind and body connection

—Keith A. Siller, MD

It is great knowing Tina. She came to me seeking a partner in her healing as she bravely fought her anxiety and other related concerns through Ayurveda. I applaud her wisdom for recognizing that it was important for her to adapt and evolve, and I honor her strength as she took the first steps toward wellness. During our work together, we embraced the teachings of Ayurveda practiced in my family in India for generations. Tina was so devoted, focused, and open to the healing that she felt more grounded and stronger after our first session.

Reawakened flows right from her heart and onto the page. It is simple and honest. You will learn how she overcame her emotional blockages, which also affected her physically. This book is full of recommendations for personal improvement and empowerment. Learn from her process, and draw your strength from her experiences.

—Dr. Manjula J. Paul, BAMS
Sound Shore Ayurveda LLC, NY

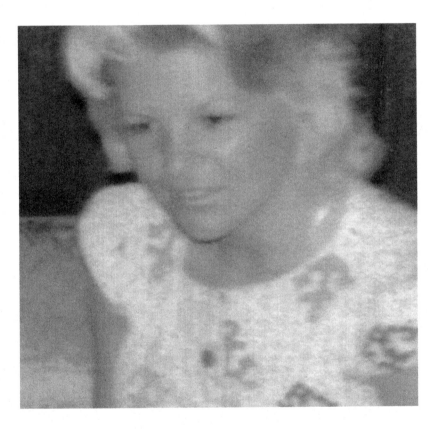

To my beautiful mother.

*The journey of a thousand miles
begins with one step.*

—Lao Tzu

Contents

Part II

– Mind –

– Body –

Acknowledgments

First and foremost, I thank my amazing husband, Mario, who supported and encouraged me in spite of all the time it took me away from him. It was a long and difficult journey for him, and I will always be so grateful for an incredible, awesome husband. I am truly blessed. My sweet dog, Cali, thank you for always putting a smile on my face.

My personal thanks to the following people; because of them, this book is a reality:

Dr. Keith Siller, Joel Harper, Dr. Manjula J. Paul, George Cerezo, Avra Blieden, Adrienne Robbins, Bob Capazzo, Lisa Armstrong, Robyn Braik, Angela Derosa, and my incredible East and West Coast family.

Behind every successful woman is a tribe of other successful women who have her back. Thank you to my fabulous girlfriends and sisters—you know who you are, and that's why I cherish you.

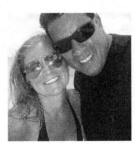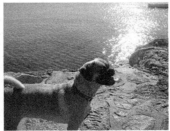

Preface

This story is about my once safe, healthy, and fully awake life that, when tragedy hit, turned upside down and became an odyssey infused with battles and tests. It took a long time to understand that the tragedy was a catalyst igniting years of personal trials for something positive. The struggles I faced ultimately proved to reawaken me.

This passage was a six-year blind journey. I ran up against the next wall barely before resolving my issues with the last. My education was boundless, and when coupled with the multitude of health and wellness solutions I worked so hard to find, I grew, suffered the next blow, beat it down, then grew again. I researched, met doctors, attended school; and each time I plummeted into illness and climbed back up, I thought it was over, but I was wrong every time. Well, almost.

Early on, I was glad to survive. As I encountered more beasts, I had to choose: Do I let these random maladies take me down, or do I tear them apart, one by one, once and for all? I dug in. I got smarter, tougher, and I set my focus. I researched holistic healers and found a course of study that ultimately inspired my career. My heart's desire shined, and my path grew more and more clear. All I learned to attain wellness, strength, and health head-to-toe set my passion afire. Once passion is ignited, there are no diversions. My sights were now set on helping others achieve their best selves. I got healthier than ever before and smarter than I ever thought I'd want to.

Eventually, I reawakened more vibrant, strong, and healthier than ever. My voyage was not easy, and I stood my ground even when I was ill. Now reawakened by all my hard-earned studies, battles, and changes, I reached my highest calling, career, and life. I felt more alive than I thought possible.

A rough patch, major crisis, or self-conflict is not a prerequisite to change or self-improvement. Wounded or well, you can take steps to reawaken to your healthiest, most vibrant self. When you are on the right path, you cannot fail; your highest self is happy and self-actualizing. When you are on the wrong path, regardless of effort, nothing feels right or seems to align in your favor. An inspired plan, goal, or unique concept doesn't mean you must immediately unravel the fibers of your current life. Start something you wish for or love to do as a hobby or a part-time job. I discovered that small consistent changes reveal new solutions and strategies on the way to big and lasting results. Grow into your best you—and your best life.

Once I got better, I got better than ever. I lived awake for a long time, but when I was put to task, I was reawakened. I wrote this book with hopes that my story and the methods and practices I used will help you reawaken to your happiest, most fulfilling life.

PART I

Introduction

When a stroke hits, every sweep of the second hand counts. But when you live in New York and your mother is having a stroke somewhere in Oregon, it's time to pray.

Time had passed since my mom and I lived a healthy, high-energy, and very physically fit life together enjoying the beaches of California. I never felt any distance between us until that horrible phone call. I had no place in my mind or heart for this possibility. She was only sixty-two. She was always healthy and active. I tried to process this biting truth, the massive slap that said my mom was gone forever. I couldn't even say good-bye. I was on my own. Abruptly. My world distorted, little misfit pieces of life drifted in and out of my mind.

Hopeless was a brand-new feeling. I was emotionally paralyzed. I was stoic. Stuck. Scared by my despair. I tried to convince myself and everyone else that I had some grief to work through; I would heal over time. That was somebody else's happy ending. My story went a different way.

That unnerving phone call stripped away my foundation, my genuine self, and my happy, balanced, and authentic life. How many times had I heard people say, "It can all change in the blink of an eye"? I never gave those words credence. Now they loomed like they were meant just for me.

Before that fateful call, my life was healthy and vibrant: up around six and out the door to walk or run with Cali, our dog, every morning. After breakfast, I was off to work. After work, I would work out. Now I reflected on that regimen in awe. Those days were gone forever; that seemed certain.

My husband, Mario, was unwavering in his understanding and support. Somehow, he was there for me through it all—and still is. I am lucky to have a very gratifying, devoted, and caring marriage with Mario, my light and my partner. Living just outside of New York City, we drove in and enjoyed dining in the city several times a week and shared many great friends and family. We walked the city together. We had a blessed, happy marriage. We never gave a moment's thought to the possibility of change.

When I lost my mom, I lost all clarity for a few years. This is my story about how I healed my life, my emotional pain, and my physical health in multiple ways, numerous times. I was physically active, vital, and highly energetic every day of my life. But one ring of a phone stole my vital self and left me ravaged with anxiety and illness.

Reawakened is about my journey and the methods and practices I learned and have incorporated for a healthy, stress-free, powerful, centered, and reawakened life. I did not learn and initiate everything at once; I spent years accumulating the methods and practices that helped me heal and grow, become well, build mental acuity, strengthen my body and my life overall, ultimately to reawaken to my greatest version of myself.

Part II of this book is designed to be accessed over time and in your own way. The applications and methods are compiled for your most convenient read and revisits.

I stayed my course no matter the situation. Some steps came naturally, others felt awkward, and then there were the experiences that tested me. I held true to personal beliefs; this single act emerged as an internal compass. By making choices based on my undeniable personal beliefs and values, the way was lit for me to meet healers who helped me get well and taught me new concepts, and each led me in unique exciting ways to my next essential step and closer to my best life.

My natural talents in organization and research also served as part of that internal compass. I used my talents as I explored the history and details of wellness, holistic healing, and dietary practices, treatment modalities, and a range of mind, body, and soul practices I now employ in my work and personal life. This is why everyone can reach their reawakened state. We are created to evolve using our gifts, talents, values, and beliefs.

Remember the internal compass in any situation but particularly when you set out to ignite your best life. To follow your calling isn't hard; all the help is there for you when you are on the right path. Do what you do best, and your passion will light the way.

You know in your heart if something is right for you. I stood my ground and did not waiver throughout my journey—to my greatest benefit as it turned out. Sometimes our inner knowing is subtle; nonetheless, we have the capacity to take the appropriate next step or a leap of faith when it is right for us. Trust your inner voice and always know that you are built to succeed in ways you will only discover if you take the next step.

I believe in keeping concepts clear and simple for the most successful and joyous life. Clutter clouds the clear view—and therefore the truth of the matter; it weighs us down with extra mental processing when we are best to be nimble, flexible, and quick to respond to opportunity. Let go! Play it smart and simple.

I wrote this book the way I live my life. My foundation is defined by one word: simplify. *This is my simple, powerful story of discovery, recovery, and ultimately being reawakened.*

The Impact

"Take me to the hospital." I forced to get the words out as I gasped for air. I couldn't breathe. I couldn't speak. Mario was driving us into the city for one of our dinners, and I was pretty sure I was having a heart attack. My heart pounded so hard, so fast; and with each passing second, it went faster. Mario tried to focus on the road, get me to a doctor quickly, and all the while watching over me.

My hands were sweating. I felt like I was right next to myself. Then I tried to hold my pulsing body still, terrified that I was about to shatter. It didn't seem like I was really there at all. I fought to get air as my heart raced on. I was so scared that I would be in heart surgery in mere minutes and possibly lose my life so young. Then I thought about my mom and was sure my fate was sealed. My eyes teared as my heart raced on; I lost all ability to make sense of things. I worried crazy worries, inventing outlandish fates for my sorry self as I gazed at my wonderful husband.

In a blink, I was in the ER with the kindest doctor. He ran several tests. I was grateful when he was done, but he surprised me with his first question. He asked if I had experienced any recent upsets or tragedies. I told him about my mother's stroke the previous month. He described the panic attack I had and how my stress and life change played a potential role. Panic attack? I thought I was going into open-heart surgery! I was thrilled with this panic attack. I was in the dark.

The doctor prescribed Valium and suggested I carry a water bottle, explaining that drinking water acts, physiologically, as a calming mechanism. His nurse said, "Panic attacks will take over your life if you let them." I pretty much felt like heart attacks will take over your life and I was leaving with my husband and a bottle of water. I was so happy I could have danced home.

Panic attacks came on out of the blue: driving to work, on the way to dinner, in elevators, even out for a peaceful walk. I tried the Valium, and it helped; but I was not comfortable with that course of treatment—I rarely take so much as an aspirin.

Solitary Confinement

Anxiety *did* take over my life. I was caged by this monster, and it was a cruel, wrathful beast, which woke me in my sleep with frightening heart palpitations and left me wrought with fear to go to sleep just the same.

I wasn't allowed my dinners with Mario; anxiety wouldn't grant that pleasure. Getting together with friends or family was off the list too. Anything beyond my front door or past my closed eyes was a giant NO. I did go to work; I forced past the barricades of anxiety and gave all I could to my full-time job, but I was always afraid to be out on my own.

Being shut in by a false sense of panic psychologically disabled me. The thought of getting in the car or walking our dog, anything I used to do without a thought was now unbearable.

I eventually made an effort, small as it was, to reach out to a few people I could speak with unguardedly. I had been absent for more than a year and had no idea what to say. I talked with family and called and met with my best of girlfriends. It's remarkable how easy words come when the person on the other end of the line clearly cares about you. I was happy I connected and felt both relief and normalcy for talking with people I loved and missed. Those were some of the first sincerely normal experiences I had in a long time.

Retaliating

This beast came to fight, and I believe we are built to fight back. One thing I urge you to adopt is the mentality that if you can understand it, you can beat it. I learned about anxiety and panic attacks—why we get them and how they work. These attacks are part of a safety mechanism called the "fight-or-flight response" that is wired into our physiological makeup from long before we left the cave. When we feel anxious, our senses kick in with the false perception of impeding threat, and we experience symptoms of fear; therefore, our physiological wiring says we must be in danger. This brings on a host of changes, some of which can affect our health. In order to increase strength and speed in anticipation of fighting or running, just some of the physical changes include the following:

- Increased blood flow to the muscles by diverting blood flow from other parts of the body, including the stomach
- Increased blood pressure, heart rate, blood sugars, and fats in order to boost energy in the body
- Increased muscle tension to provide the body with extra speed and strength

Thus when an anxiety attack comes on, our body sends blood away from the midsection to the head for quick thinking to the arms and legs to enable us to flee, and our digestion shuts down.

I moved on armed with a better understanding of what anxiety made me think ("If I feel fear, there must be danger"), what anxiety was doing to my body (tearing down my digestive system), and lastly, what it was doing to my life (entrapping me, keeping me from my daily workouts and dining with Mario).

In Part II, my first topic is anxiety and panic attacks. There I offer multiple techniques to win the battle and take your life back from the beast called Anxiety.

I wanted to take a holistic route to healing and learned that beyond mind-body therapies of meditation and yoga and the practice of natural remedies such as herbs blended and prescribed for health reasons, the host of complementary and alternative medical avenues was vast. It would require more strength before I tackled this important goal.

Working out was something I could do from home, and I felt ready to get started. My good friend and longtime personal trainer, George, was willing to help. I had the blessings of good people like George throughout my battles. It only takes one kind person to get you to the next step, and I was blessed in that way.

George signed on for a few days each week. He modified my workouts to exercise different muscle groups and rebuild my strength and endurance over time. A few months later, I started to feel more like myself.

I also practiced a four-part breathing sequence every morning that helped center me for my day and was a good anxiety buster. This sequence is outlined in Part II.

My panic attacks devastated me for over a year. As I loosened the chains of anxiety, I was hit with food allergies, and my strength and digestive system deteriorated further.

Where was the energetic, effervescent, and highly capable woman I used to be? Who was this dull, fragile shell of a human into whom I slowly was crumbling?

The Search for
a Solution

I started seeing an acupuncturist but was not comfortable with the needles. I moved on to reflexology, massage therapy, and nutrition counseling. I tried to rework my mind and body from the inside out and vice versa. Each try was like those waterproof Band-Aids that come off in the swimming pool; I wanted something that would really stick, and for me, no therapy felt genuine and lasting to my body and issues. More work was clearly ahead.

Avra, a friend of mine, eventually recommended Adrienne, a holistic healthcare professional. By the time I met with her, I was riddled with frustration. When the first step was paperwork, I pushed with my last drop of energy to continue. Feeling weak and ill made formalities tough. I suffered every line, every box, on every page, through each form. Then I found journaling each bite of food for two weeks was next. The thought was exhausting. Tedious activities overwhelmed me. However, I held my referral in high regard, and she knew my issues. I held faith that Adrienne could help if she was fully apprised of my issues and challenges. Through my malaise, I scribed each bite for the next two weeks.

With data in hand, Adrienne ultimately diagnosed my food allergies, but not the ones I thought I had. She also established that I had a weakened immune system. With my health in her hands, everything I took going forward was natural, which gave me great comfort. Every week, I felt stronger and more focused.

Getting well happens in phases. As I felt well, more often than not, I started joining my friends for a dinner. I joined my family more often, and I returned to some of my other normal routines.

New life pulsed through me each day as I woke at 6:00 a.m. and ran with Cali again. To be out in the morning air, in the rich splendor of nature, and witness the day surge with energy was an enormous gift.

Mario and I began to travel, which we always loved. We hit up one of our favorite islands, Bermuda, and other equally sunny beaches, and overnighted in Philadelphia, Boston, Rhode Island, and so many sweet little towns boasting with shops, pubs, and fun dining locales. It was always so nice to bond with my amazing husband on those trips. He truly is the love of my life and has supported me through so much. I was excited to be able to share a level love playing field in those beautiful cities. My heart yearned for these getaways for so long. It was absolute heaven on earth.

I am also blessed with an irreplaceable friendship circle. When I finally reconnected live and in person with those fabulous ladies to rekindle such special friendships, that was my special therapy. This is my go-to group for absolutely everything under the sun. We chat and laugh until it hurts whenever we gather. But if any one of us needs anything any time, we are there for each other—for life.

My life was coming together in all areas. I was on cloud nine, and most of the time it was hard to remember just how miserable I had been; I was too enthralled with every wonderful moment.

New York City seems limitless, and I have always made an effort to enjoy the wealth of opportunities it offers. Before I got sick, I never missed much. Now Mario and I were back to the city for brunch, dinner, or a sweet and tender walk together on the West Side Highway.

I returned to rollerblading—yes, I rollerblade! You don't have to wear rainbow socks to rollerblade; you just have to bring your spirit and expect a good time. Try it! I have rollerbladed in many areas including beautiful Central Park and of course the West Side Highway.

I was thrilled with my excellent health. My workout schedule was back to a daily selection of fun options, and I participated in fitness events for a great cause in the city. Freedom from anxiety and the sense of power that came with such hard-earned wellness was a reward I accepted with my sights set on doing all I could to catch up on the life I had missed. Mostly, though, I felt I had finally landed, and that feeling warmed my soul and made me feel like dancing.

Déjà Vu

I enjoyed two symptom-free years. I forgot all about illness and had fun. One day I couldn't take a deep breath. My lungs felt heavy. My stomach was sick.

For the next three months, I endured one doctor after the next, suggesting I was "coming down with something" or "it was something I ate." Recommendations came up empty: "take an antacid," "eat a bland diet," and so it went as I remained ill and drained of energy. An upper endoscopy eventually pointed to gastritis.

Along with gastritis, I began to struggle again with a compromised immune system. I wanted to control my meal contents and preparation to try to protect my system. We stayed in, and most of the time I cooked.

My immune system was compromised for over a year. My overall disease ate at everything. It ate at my immune system. It ate at my stomach, my schedule, my sense of reality. One thing after another came apart, and I couldn't get anything in my world under control.

The Light Bulb

It was then that I had an epiphany. I wanted the education in holistic wellness that would give me the knowledge, background, and education to choose my own foods and really know what is right for me. It was the right time for me to dig in and learn as much as I could. Avra had a history in health and wellness. She introduced me to health coaching; she had strong feelings about my potential in the field, which I am now grateful she shared. She also introduced me to the Institute for Integrative Nutrition (IIN). I dove in and learned all that I could about the school. I was immediately drawn, from deep in my heart, to the path of serving as a health coach.

My experience with a compromised immune system equally inspired me to study at the institute. Their extensive curriculum contained the kinds of topics and areas of study that meant so much to me by this point. I was most intrigued by the depth at which the school focused on food and health issues. Their comprehensive information looked like it might cover lasting solutions to heal my digestive issues and other holistic pathways for my other issues.

Although I was not yet at my best, I thought that along with the variety of dietary theories, it would benefit me to hear the impressive list of speakers and absorb the stimulating information about health and living well. It sounded intriguing, and I dared to believe that with so many sources of information, I could get on the path to wellness.

Through my IIN studies, I learned many helpful things—diverse and valuable, highly applicable information that I will apply throughout my personal and professional life. One key newer finding that I invested in and is now scientifically backed is bio-individuality. The premise is that each person is biologically individual, thus the term bio-individuality. It is based on the understanding that every human being's metabolism, food tolerance makeup, and so on is unique. No two people are alike; thus no single diet or protocol is appropriate for any mass of people. Bio-individuality offers a unique, customizable approach.

Part II provides detailed discussions on health coaching, bio-individuality, and other keys to building a healthy, calm, fit, and highly satisfying life. With a commitment to be more vital, happier, and living a more balanced life, it is possible for anyone to see rich results across all areas of their life.

It was at the Institute for Integrative Nutrition that I also learned about the Paleo diet. This diet is a popular choice for autoimmune issues and many other complications. It is discussed in Part II. While I was educating myself on the dietary theories, my husband and I tried a lot of them, but we always returned to the Paleo diet.

Full Throttle

The Paleo diet is still part of our everyday life, but if we go out to an event, our diet will change. I love food too much to be on any diet consistently. So long as I am eating clean and enjoying incredible, high-level energy, I am more than pleased. I also did a lot of research and trial and error, which helped me to recover. Knowledge is the key to health and wellness. I am grateful to have had the opportunity to study at the Institute for Integrative Nutrition.

After six months on the Paleo diet, my immune system was improving. Meanwhile, Adrienne, my holistic healer had treated my gastritis. I decided to make some small modifications while continuing to eat clean: I ate whole, natural, unprocessed foods. I eliminated soy, dairy, gluten, and wheat from my diet to avoid immune-based food reactions. Eliminating all processed foods and clean eating seemed to have a powerful effect on me and my immune system.

Once I completed rather extensive research, I found these reads particularly inspiring: Joshua Rosenthal's *Integrative Nutrition*, davidji's *Secrets of Meditation: A Practical Guide to Inner Peace and Personal Transformation* (this book details a variety of meditation styles, which were easy to follow), David Wolfe's *Superfoods* (a fairly quick study that I could apply immediately for higher energy and reduced stress), and you guessed it, *The Secret*, which should be on everyone's list.

Also, *10% Happier* is a book on meditation that strongly resonated with me. Author Dan Harris talks to the novice meditator. I recommend this book to those wanting the benefit of meditation but looking for help getting started. Meditation is something that seems impossible until one day it clicks, and you have the understanding. Stay with it; if you are trying to meditate, you will get there. In Part II, I share my start with meditation, provide guidance on getting started, and offer some helpful resources.

With a focus on self-healing, I explored an ancient practice called Ayurveda. I had heard of it long ago and hoped it might hold something meaningful for me. The Ayurvedic platform is to treat the individual. Every individual is unique; thus no diet or lifestyle routine will be effective for all patients. Ayurveda aims to bring us back to our true constitution and restore balance in our bodies and minds. Food and lifestyle routines are the primary medicines. Part II includes a full segment on Ayurveda.

My search for an Ayurvedic doctor led to the impressive, prestigious Dr. Manjula J. Paul, BAMS (Bachelor of Ayurvedic Medicine and Surgery). In my first session, Dr. Paul performed a pulse analysis, which is often the most significant first step. She also conducted a personalized lifestyle assessment, which covered nutritional counseling, herbal medication, body therapies, skin care, aromatherapy, and exercise specified for my unique system and issues. I also received material on daily and seasonal routines applicable to my sensitivities.

It was intriguing to receive so much personalized guidance. This is the standard by which Ayurvedic practitioners and doctors operate. Ayurveda is distinct and exclusive by any comparison. Your guidance will suit you and will be comfortable for you to achieve. A guided assessment is a personable, happy experience. As you progress, your life will open to improved health, more energy, and countless benefits that suit you for any mental or physical issue.

I didn't know what to expect from Ayurveda or from Dr. Paul. Afterward, I was relaxed and honestly felt better than ever. I was well! I was beyond well—I had finally evolved to my new self, my balanced, happy, focused self. I did not need a monthly Ayurvedic consultation, but I built it into my routine because it made me feel so wonderful.

It wasn't one thing that launched my wellness; it was the journey and my unrelenting effort to get well. I never imagined I would evolve past returning to the awake person I was prior to losing my mom. Ultimately, I reawakened to my best, most vital self and stepped into my new life, my life calling—helping others using a wide variety of research, experience, and the vast applications and education that comes with a health coach certification. I embraced my journey of research, classes, and learning through new and ancient studies. I was reawakened fresh, bright, filled with vigor, and new vision. I have no reason to let up; my passion is set afire!

PART II

Introduction

My mission is to serve as a coach to my clients with a shared goal of achieving a happy life of health and wellness. My work incorporates much of the guidance that is the basis for this book. I believe in the Ayurvedic principles and practices: each individual is unique; therefore, treatment must be equally unique. My focus with each client includes lifestyle, diet, body energies, and other targeted and specific life and health needs.

In this section, I offer a variety of practices, guidance, and information to enhance your amazing life and to flesh out what was only touched on in Part I. Try something now and bookmark something else for a while later. Learn and grow. I took years to learn all of this, so take your time too.

Whatever you do with the information in this section, don't be too quick to pass it by. We tend to discover the practices we respond to best by giving them a try. Be open. You might surprise yourself—I did!

Look for groups in your area that either practice (such as yoga, qigong, or meditation) or hold discussions (such as Ayurveda) on topics you find interesting. Online research is popular, but watch out for advertisements and unknown individuals posting less-than-complete, inaccurate material. Look for associations and other reputable sources. Consider picking up a few books on a topic that interests you; peruse the Resources at the end of this book.

Regardless of how you follow on from here, I hope you simply do follow on. Consider bringing a friend or two along with you; it makes attending a class or picking up new studies and practices much more fun, memorable, and fulfilling. And friends keep each other going, which is a great benefit of having wonderful friends.

MIND

The mind is everything.
What you think you become.
- Buddha -

Anxiety and Panic Attacks

Take over anxiety before it takes over you.

This section provides some of the tips, tricks, and solutions that have helped me resolve or control anxiety and/or panic attacks.

The Anxiety Trick and How to Beat It

During an anxiety attack, we experience shortness of breath, our muscles tense, heart races, and stomach feels ill. All of these and more physical responses are *real* measurable reactions. The onset of panic or anxiety is medically noted. What happens after the onset is between you and anxiety; one of you will win.

Anxiety has been caught at its devious little game, "The Anxiety Trick," and it puts you in an "if-then" scenario: "*If* I feel fear, *then* I am in danger." So to beat anxiety at its own trick, stay aware that there is no danger. Realize that while you feel an onset of anxiety, it will leave if you do not react to the false sensations it stirs. If you fight, struggle, and release control, anxiety wins by making you behave as if danger lurks. When you feel anxiety starting up, keep it real, as described in the upcoming tip, "Get Real and Get Calm," and take your power back from that trickster anxiety.

To help ensure you win the game against anxiety, master the following easy breathing methods; they will keep calm from slipping away.

It is a medical fact that if an exhale is longer than an inhale, the body will relax. Simply inhale to a count of about four (or a count that is comfortable and natural for you), then exhale slowly so you are able to exhale for a longer count, say about six or seven (you will choose your count). Even one pass at this relaxes the body. This can be done in public just as easily as privately with ideal results toward peace.

The other breathing method is an alteration to how you exhale. Your counts remain the same; however, during the exhale, draw your lips around an invisible straw, then blow out your exhale. The limitation of airflow created by your "straw" extends the exhale—you are able to control, maintain, and expand the length of the exhale incrementally. Nothing feels so calming as the smooth flow of an exhale that ushers out irritations, issues, pain, or confusion through that "straw."

Taking some key concepts from this segment, a better night's sleep is also at hand. Regardless of a racing mind that causes muscles to pulse and become tense or simply a general state of uneasiness, difficulty sleeping tends to affect most of us from time to time.

Perform the same breathing exercise (without the straw) ensuring your exhale runs longer than your inhale. Enjoy your body's now calm, relaxed state. Additionally, note the position of your head: is your chin angled forward or upward? This incites a learned physiological response. Head up means be alert and ready, the day is at hand. Tip your head just slightly down to elicit the response to rest safely; your mind and body react by slipping into a restful state, ready to sleep and recharge.

Stay Hydrated

Almost every function of the body is managed by and related to the efficient flow of water through our system. Water transports hormones, chemical messengers, and nutrients to vital organs of the body. If the body is not kept well hydrated, a variety of signals, such as anxiety, are likely to be triggered. The standard guidelines recommend we drink eight glasses of water daily for general health. Carrying a bottle of water with you is a smart way to keep anxiety at bay.

Did you ever forget to eat and start feeling shaky and panicky? That's those cells talking!

Get Real and Get Calm

You can quell even the worst state of panic, wherever you might be, by refocusing on your surroundings instead of allowing your physiological response carry your attack to greater heights.

Take control of your breath; be sure you are not taking in more oxygen than your body can process: slow your exhale as you breathe, then begin to breathe deeper. While it is ideal to be seated in any comfortable position and place, you can perform this easy, effective process standing, leaning, and anywhere you might be.

Focus on only one item; don't be concerned about everything else around you. In your mind, or aloud, begin to describe it in detail. Be clear and specific. Don't move on to another object until you have completely detailed the first one: "I am looking across the table at my cell phone. It is face-up. It has a glass face; there are no new messages because that icon is not lit. I see the edges of the case are worn. The bottom edges are more worn than the top edges (be incredibly detailed); it is a silver-colored case. The case has a beaded pattern, etc." Move on only after completely exhausting the description of your initial item. "Now I see my running shoes. I just bought them last month. They are white with black accents (describe the accents). The shoe strings are gray." You are providing your mind and body with your true reality.

The fact that there is nothing to fear becomes clear throughout your being: your mind and physiologic system will calm. This process happens quite fast if you keep focus on one item so that your brain recognizes that what you are busying yourself with is your full reality. Your focus on the ordinary—the truth—will succeed.

Be Calm with Bananas

Bananas are loaded with potassium and vitamin B-6 to quickly calm the nervous system. Former Miss Universe Olivia Culpo says, "When I was competing in Miss Universe and Miss USA, I always ate a banana before going on stage. It's been my trick to settle nerves since I was little." Also, if you cannot sleep, a half of a banana is a healthy solution.

Other Benefits of Bananas

General benefits: Overcome depression due to high levels of tryptophan, which convert into serotonin; protect against type II diabetes; aid weight loss; strengthen the nervous system; help with the production of white blood cells; relieve anemia with added iron—FDA recognized for their high potassium and low salt benefits—able to lower blood pressure and protect against heart attack and stroke; rich in pectin to aid in digestion and gently chelate toxins and heavy metals from the body.

Gastrointestinal benefits: Act as a prebiotic to stimulate growth of friendly bacteria in the bowel and produce digestive enzymes to assist in absorbing nutrients; help normalize bowel activity and end constipation; restore electrolytes; soothe the digestive tract; natural antacid to relieve heartburn, acid reflux, and GERD; help relieve stomach ulcers by coating the stomach lining against corrosive acids.

Preventative benefits: Prevent kidney cancer, protect eyes against macular degeneration, high in antioxidants (thus they protect the body from free radicals and chronic disease), reduce nausea from morning sickness, ward off binging by controlling blood sugar, and relieve stress by regulating blood sugar.

Four-Part Deep Breathing

A Daily Stressbuster

Before I adopted mindful meditation, which I now practice every morning, I started each day with this breathing sequence. Four-Part Deep Breathing helped me a great deal during my toughest year of battling panic and anxiety.

I find that Four-Part Deep Breathing is a healthy way to start the day and a great way to maintain power over stress, anxiety, or fear. It's beneficial to kick off the day relaxed and stress-free. If you cannot take time to release stress and do a breathing exercise first thing, keep Four-Part Deep Breathing in mind anytime you feel constriction or anxiety.

You can do this seated upright with or without legs folded or lying on your back. Be sure you are not hunched over; you want your breath to reach deep into your lungs and your diaphragm (tummy area). To be sure you are sitting properly, imagine there is a string that comes up from the floor, runs straight up your spine, and along the back of your head. You want that string to be nice and long and straight. You can reach your right arm up and then drop your hand straight down behind your head. Pull the imaginary string. This will help you sit even straighter, open your hips more, and open up your chest. Now you are very well set to take some nice deep breaths!

Close your eyes gently and inhale deeply, intently, to the count of four; then hold to the count of four. Next, consciously exhale to the count of four and hold to the count of four. Repeat a few times. If you feel anxious and it is affecting your stomach, breathe into your stomach. If your heart is racing, focus your breath directly into that area as you do this exercise pay close attention to your exhale, imagining the slow, controlled release of anxiety.

Boost Your Brain Power

Do the write thing.

Slide that keyboard aside and leave the Kindle at home; it's time to fire up those neurons! I would open every one of the upcoming segments by asking you to journal if I didn't know better. Writing by hand has such a massive positive impact I am surprised we don't see more articles popping up to support it. Then I realize nobody's going to blast this important information on their e-zine, blog, or any social media where we get our information these days. Luckily, books still have a place in the world; and speaking of, here's a short list of famous folks who still pen their films and books by hand:

- The prolific author of books such as *Blonde* and *them*, Joyce Carol Oates prefers to write everything longhand, for up to eight hours a day. In an interview with *Salon*, she said, "Why is this so unusual? Every writer has written by hand until relatively recent times. Writing is a consequence of thinking, planning, dreaming. This is the process that results in writing, rather than the way in which the writing is recorded."
- Director Quentin Tarantino writes his own screenplays in pen and paper. "My ritual is I never use a typewriter or computer. I just write it all by hand. I go to a stationery store and buy a notebook. I just buy one and then fill it up. I buy a bunch felt pens, and I'm like, 'These are the

pens I'm going to write *Grindhouse* with,'" he said in an interview with *Reuters*.

- Author Amy Tan prefers to write early drafts longhand, saying that she loves the act of physical writing. "Writing by hand helps me remain open to all those particular circumstances, all those little details that add up to the truth," she said in an interview with *The Atlantic*.
- Neil Gaiman is a sci-fi jack of all trades who prefers to write his novels by hand.
- Tom Wolfe, the famous author of *The Bonfire of the Vanities*, wrote his 2012 novel *Back to Blood* entirely by longhand.
- Wayne Dyer, Ph.D., an internationally renowned author and speaker in self-development has written thirty books, entirely with pen and paper. In a recent blog, he shared, "I just let the ideas flow through my heart. I don't write with a machine."

Writing can be highly creative, extremely calming, and for many, a problem-solving process. One great thing about a pen and paper is that no matter what the problem or issue, once it's on paper, it is out of your mind. You now own it rather than it owning you. This might seem odd and perhaps not even worth the bother, but it is tremendously effective. When we write, we solve problems. Whether working through the entire issue in one session or journaling, many areas of the brain are engaged that otherwise are not part of the process. It feels good because it is good. If you feel panic or high stress, it can melt away in just minutes with a pen and paper.

If you want to journal but don't know what to write, grab a notebook and a pen and start with, "I don't know what to write." Write about how new this feels. Just write and don't stop. You will find great joy and therapy in writing if you invest a bit of time.

The next section offers some of the biggest ways that writing by hand can help our brains, provided by Dr. Marc Seifer, a graphologist and handwriting expert.

Writing a calming sentence is a form of graphotherapy, Seifer says. Jotting a sentence like, "I will be more peaceful" twenty times per day can have an impact for anyone, especially those with attention deficit disorder. "This actually calms the person and retrains the brain." Also, writing anything in cursive can coordinate the left and right brain.

It also inspires creativity. Taking pen to paper inspires more creative thought because it is a slower process than just typing something on a keyboard, Seifer says. Also, I suggest that you make your goals and to-do lists by hand. As you write, more areas of your brain are engaged, and if you have done this in the past, you might have noticed that the list becomes more precise. Your memory and creative thought process, which works through the project, kicks in; recall goes up; and those little extras like shower soap or a few gardening supplies make it onto the list—or you might realize that certain items for a project needed rethinking.

Goals in particular are best written by hand because while you are crafting your goals, your brain provides the details that give you an edge. As you write, problems get solved. This also allows you to draft a few mini-goals that can be accomplished more quickly. The ability to strike a line through some goals sooner leads to that sense of accomplishment we all need to spur us on. When your next project strikes, grab a pen and paper!

Lastly, writing sharpens aging minds. Some physicians claim that the act of writing—which engages motor skills, memory, and more—is a good cognitive exercise for baby boomers who want to keep their minds sharp as they age. The linked regions of the brain are activated while writing by hand, but not while typing or texting. In short, writing works the brain muscle like nothing else—for every age.

So engage your brain. Write in your journal, thank-you and holiday cards, shopping lists, and goals. The more you write, the better!

Have Vision

If you see it in your life, you will have it.

Most have read the book or seen the self-help, motivational film *The Secret*. In it, one speaker discusses his Vision Board, which is a popular tool that people use to place extra focus, energy, and intent on the outcomes most desired in their lives. Based on the Law of Attraction, a Vision Board can be useful in realizing dreams, goals, and successes.

For instance, if a woman is single and deeply wishes to marry, she might paste or pin a picture of a wedding ring or wedding gown on her board. Let's say she also would like to vacation on an island during her time off. Expect to see an image of an island or people walking seaside.

So a Vision Board is a collage of images, objects, pictures, and affirmations of your dreams, goals, intents, outcomes, and things that will make you happy. You want this board to be your vision of what you want to come into your life. If you want to be a leader of something big, make it your vision and intent, but view your board frequently and believe deeply. That energetic connection makes your vision clear to the Universe, puts you on the right path, and aligns you with your dreams.

I look at my Vision Board each morning, and I carry a photo of it on my phone so I can glance at it on occasions. The greater your intent, the better the response. It isn't a magic trick. Intend on having that thing, being in that career, or having that outcome. Intent is the key to everything with a Vision Board and when connecting with a greater source.

To make a Vision Board, you need a large piece of cardboard, whether it is cut from a box or purchased from an office supply store. Tape or paste images from magazines, photos, anything that represents what you most want. Cut out headlines and write out affirmations, use any method you wish to attach statements to your images, or let the statements represent your wishes. There is no wrong way to build a Vision Board. You are aligning with the Universe and intending your happiest outcomes. The Universe operates on yes or no. Now you must place your order.

TINA'S BOARD

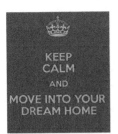

KEEP CALM AND MOVE INTO YOUR DREAM HOME

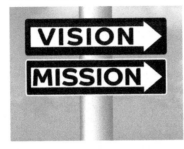

VISION ▶
MISSION ▶

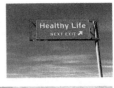

Healthy Life NEXT EXIT

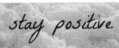

stay positive

Do more for mom's cause

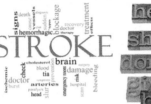

STROKE

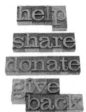

help share donate give back

MOVE INTO MY BEACH HOUSE

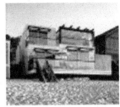

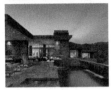

ATTEND A YOGA RETREAT

Become a Certified Health Coach

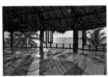

HAVE CALI SWIM IN THE OCEAN

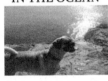

COACHING

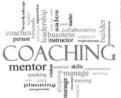

live in the moment

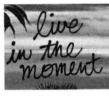

KEEP CALM AND SEEK A HEALTH COACH

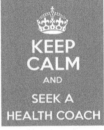

ATTEND
SECRETS OF MEDITATION & AYURVEDA WORKSHOP

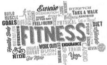

FITNESS

RYS 200 yoga ALLIANCE

YOGA

CERTIFIED davidji Masters of Wisdom & Meditation TEACHER

© Can Stock Photo

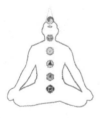

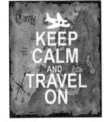

KEEP CALM AND TRAVEL ON

ALOHA

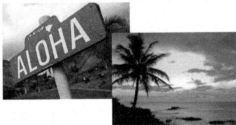

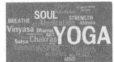

BECOME A CERTIFIED AYURVEDIC PRATITIONER

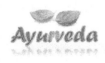

Ayurveda

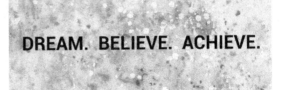

DREAM. BELIEVE. ACHIEVE.

Mindful Meditation
Let go, yes you can do it.

Introduction

This is how I learned to meditate. I took a six-week class, and I let myself go through the process.

I tried. I sat, eyes closed, legs folded, and slowly inhaled, then pushed all the negativity and toxicity out as I exhaled. With each breath, I made the effort to drop into a deeper state of peace. Then I would think about the negative stuff and keep thinking and not let go. I am a Type A. We tend to be dialed up to about an eight, and meditation is a wonderful place where your vibration is at perhaps a two or three. I stayed with it; I don't give up.

Slowly my mind and body began to learn. As my understanding grew, I felt good instead of feeling like I was working hard. I didn't just breathe deeply, I breathed into me... into my heart, which needed healing; my gut, which had taken so many hits along the way; my mind, which was growing and changing. I understood the depth of that breath. When I blew out, I blew out hurt and the pain of the past and all kinds of pieces of my journey that needed to be released. This gave me the ability to settle in and go deeper. That was what meditation began to mean for me. And I could express gratitude for this healing.

I began to be in the moment. This is a life practice called mindfulness, and those who achieve it live their lives in the moment—an exceptionally healthy, peaceful way to live. For now, I was just so pleased to be in the moment during meditation. I was beginning a transformation that was far more than this one single conquest, but it had to start here. I had to be able to hear my true self and release all the hard things, sad things, pressure, and I have to say, primarily the things that were outside of me that I was allowing in and letting hurt or stop me.

Almost nobody in our current times enters meditation without hitting some rough spots. Don't be discouraged; let your body learn to let go and give over to your mind. Let your mind learn that it is safe to set free, float, see past darkness. If I could get there, you can too. On the following pages, I describe mindful meditation and offer a meditation for beginners along with a meditation journal.

To get a sense of mindfulness meditation, try one of Dr. Ronald Siegel's guided recordings. They are available at no charge at www. mindfulness-solution.com. davidji offers guided meditations and a host of meditation information at davidji.com.
Additional resources are available at the back of this book.

Mindful Meditation Explained

Meditation helps improve concentration, mental clarity, emotional positivity, and offers a calm, truthful lens through which one views the nature of things. One popular mindful meditation is mindfulness of breath. Breath awareness steadies the mind so it can delve deeper into meditation and not wander into other thought. Breath is the only thing to which your mind holds focus. Any other thought is acknowledged and dismissed.

I investigated meditation to treat my anxiety. I kept a thirty-day meditation journal for extra encouragement. Reading, educational videos, classes, and workshops led me to mindful meditation. Both qigong (discussed next) and meditation have reduced my anxiety and helped heal my immune system.

Now that I have conquered my anxiety, I practice a morning meditation and qigong two to three times per week. Individuals who incorporate meditation into their lives resolve problems, release tension, and come out of a meditative state refreshed. Oftentimes it is suggested by counselors as part of a variety of treatments.

Meditation should be done at a time of day when you can truly invest. Maybe this is three o'clock in your office or just after you arrive home for the day. To start your day with mindful meditation is effective because it sets your mind, body, and the brain itself into a mode of peace, well-being, and universal connection. You will start with learning to focus on your breath and releasing. As you adapt, you will begin to understand the ability to connect at a broader level. Often this is easier to do if you are in a meditation class. It feels comforting, and I have found it helpful, over time, to wire my thinking and behavior to a bigger source of both kindness and access for help and wisdom. It is a beautiful goal.

Basic Meditation for Beginners

There are no rules in meditation. Whatever you experience during this mindful breathing meditation is right for you.

Upon waking, I turn on lights to trigger wakefulness, then sit cross-legged on my meditation cushion for eight minutes (my lucky number is eight) and meditate. For me, a morning meditation sets the tone for the day. Here are some easy steps for breathing meditation:

1. Sit in an easy cross-legged or comfortable position. I use a meditation cushion. Cushions designed for meditation practice include zafus, gomdens, and meditation cushions. You might use a folded blanket or another kind of cushion or bench. Be sure you are relaxed and supported.

2. Close your eyes or focus on one spot or light a candle and focus on the flame. Commit to a relaxed state of stillness.

3. Do nothing to control your breath; breathe naturally.

4. Roll your shoulders slowly forward, then slowly back.

5. Let your head fall gently toward your left shoulder, then toward your right shoulder. Do not force or strain your neck, only relax.

6. Let your muscles relax.

7. Note how your body moves with each inhalation and exhalation. Observe your chest, shoulders, rib cage, and belly. Make no effort to control your breath; simply bring it to your attention. If your mind wonders off into thoughts, pull it back. It is the nature of thoughts to take your attention away from your focus. Thoughts take you to the past or future, worries or dreams. If your mind drifts, acknowledge the thought and let it go. Your subconscious mind will hold it for you to tend to later. Gently bring your attention back to your breath.

Maintain this mindful meditation for eight minutes, and then try it for ten, fifteen, and work toward twenty minutes. Have a sincere moment of gratitude when you're finished—you will learn about being grateful the more you meditate. At first, when coming out of your meditative state, simply rest your face into a gentle smile as you breathe into awareness. Be grateful for that moment.

The more you meditate, the greater your wisdom. The greater your wisdom, the greater your awareness. As your awareness is enriched, so your gratitude will grow.

Journaling over the next thirty days is richly rewarding, whether you write daily or every few days. Record thoughts, feelings, things that might happen in life and how you approach or handle them and so on. It's *your* journal; write what comes to *your* mind. Perhaps you will journal new ideas or even sketch once in a while. There are no rules to journaling, and journals are a wonderful outlet for all things. A simple notebook at your bedside can become one of your best new practices.

Benefits of Meditation:

- Decreased anxiety, reduced stress
- Lower heart rate
- Lower blood pressure
- Improved focus, concentration, and productivity
- Improved blood circulation
- Increased sense of well-being, deeper relaxation
- Greater compassion, increased gratitude
- Heightened awareness of that which truly matters

The benefits of meditation cannot be contained. Everyone receive based on their life, personality, needs, focus, commitment, and unique personal being.

30 Day Meditation Journal

Day 1

Day 2

Day 3

Day 4

Day 5

Day 6

Day 7

Day 8

Day 9

Day 10

Day 11

Day 12

Day 13

Day 14

Day 15

Notes:

30 Day Meditation Journal

Day 16

Day 17

Day 18

Day 19

Day 20

Day 21

Day 22

Day 23

Day 24

Day 25

Day 26

Day 27

Day 28

Day 29

Day 30 - Congratulations!

Notes:

Qigong
Let it flow

Qigong (pronounced chi gung) is a Chinese word meaning "life energy cultivation" and is a mind-body exercise for health and healing, meditation, and martial arts. I discovered qigong while searching for ways to strengthen my immune system. I took a class and loved the way I felt afterward; I continued practicing on my own. At the end of this discussion is a broad list of benefits qigong offers.

Qigong incorporates slow and meaningful body movement, inner focus, and regulated breathing. Mindfulness is integrated: this means living in the moment (not focusing on the past, which is over, or the future, which is only a postulation). Awareness of the moment proceeds in a nonreactive, peaceful, nonjudgmental, and open-hearted way.

Understanding your qi (chi) as the essential, vital force between *body* (matter, structure) and *mind* (process, function) helps in sensing illnesses or disease within your body. As you practice qigong, moving mindfully, you will naturally work into areas in need of healing.

To comprehend the physical, emotional, spiritual, and healing impact of qigong, taichi, or yoga, it should be experienced firsthand. Anybody, including me, writing of these beautiful practices with so many benefits will never capture what you will feel and know by doing. The mind-body connection is one of the biggest differences between Eastern and Western healing. Eastern healing works to create an unblocked flow through the entire individual: mind and body are inseparable.

Qi, or chi, in its most basic meaning is *life force* and is treated as energy. Qigong and taichi (and acupuncture) improve physical and mental energy by opening blocked channels within the mind and body so that energy runs efficiently. A body that is ill has lower energy because there is a block in the energy flow. Blockages can be nearly anywhere and cannot be covered in this book, but a few examples include posture, tendons, flexibility, muscle tension, and respiratory issues. (See the list of benefits at the end of this article.) Unblocking what may need healing improves the energy flow and leads to health and vitality. This includes increased mental energy, making one a higher producer, with more mental stamina, ideas, and creativity. Mood and mental illnesses can also open and be healed. Spiritual energy improves as well.

After my first qigong class, I purchased *Qigong for Beginners* by Chris Pei, a DVD that makes a great addition to anyone's routine once they have experienced a live class. The only way to know if qigong could be your practice awaiting discovery is to take a class. I liked qigong for its interplay of concentrated slow movement and meditation. People tend to relate strongly with qigong or yoga and other such practices because they tried a beginner's class and connected with that particular practice. It will happen for you as well, and it happens quickly.

Finding the right class and classmates is key. Would you go to any hair dresser? Random doctors? Your qigong practitioner will assist you in connecting mind and body, then guide you as you learn about the practice. You might be very happy with the first class you attend, but if you are unhappy, don't give up the practice when perhaps it is the classroom or your connection with the teacher that needs modifying.

Benefits of Qigong

Qigong practitioners tend to live a long life.
Builds power ⁼ Improves flexibility
Increases balance ⁼ Improves posture
Loosens the muscles ⁼ Prevents joint injury
Aids digestion ⁼ Lowers stress
Improves blood sugar levels ⁼ Lowers blood pressure
Improves circulation ⁼ Reduces stroke risk
Strengthens organs ⁼ Lowers heart rate ⁼ Normalizes EKG
Slows respiration ⁼ Improves asthma
Rebuilds the immune system ⁼ Relieves bronchitis
Helps kidney function ⁼ Builds bone density
Balances emotions ⁼ Relieves Migraines ⁼ Strengthens nerves
Destroys free radicals ⁼ Fosters skin elasticity
Strengthens ligaments ⁼ Averts muscle spasms
Increases injury recovery ⁼ Reduces pain
Addresses early senility ⁼ Improves Memory
Normalizes sex hormone levels ⁼ Can correct impotence and frigidity

BODY

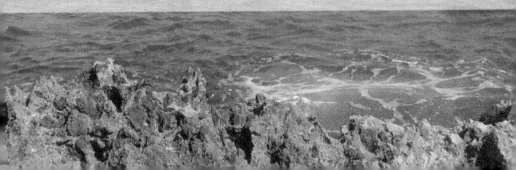

The greatest wealth is health.
- Virgil -

What Is a Health Coach?

Let's get started!

Health coaching is a relatively new profession. Put simply, it is the idea of "not just nutrition, but lifestyle management," says Deepak Chopra. A health coach deals with a rather comprehensive spectrum of how human beings operate: the benefit of food when absorbed in combinations, the impact on the mind, body, decision-making, and lifestyle during shifts or changes such as stress, love, money, and so on.

Goals include educating and coaching clients to rise to a more inspired and informed lifestyle, empowering them to make life choices that lead to health, rather than curbing disease, and guiding them toward overall wellness and comfort. A health coach is successful when their client is making consistent modifications for a lifetime of results.

I received my certification as a health coach from the Institute for Integrative Nutrition (IIN). It is my greatest passion to help people rise to be their best version of themselves. I employ the innovative coaching methods I studied at the IIN, along with so much of what I am sharing throughout this book. It is exciting and rewarding to assist clients in their journey to wellness in multiple facets of their lives.

I am versed in practical lifestyle management techniques and over one hundred dietary theories. Some of the key diet theories I found valuable include ayurveda, gluten-free, paleo, raw, vegan, and macrobiotics. I also found the extensive cutting-edge knowledge in holistic nutrition and preventative approaches to wellness to be crucial to coaching.

Among the studies I most value is a scientifically proven program called bio-individuality. Simply put, the premise is that each person is *biologically individual,* thus the term. It is based on the understanding that every human being's metabolism, food tolerance makeup, lifestyle, and so on are unique. No two people are alike; thus no one diet or protocol is appropriate. Bio-individuality offers a unique, customizable approach to diet and nutrition. It also explains why fad diets tend to fail—for a short time, a diet can cause a certain metabolic response, but over time, each body will make up for that "trick" or nutritional adjustment.

The Paleo Diet

I tried many of the dietary theories I studied at the Institute for Integrative Nutrition, and the one I continually returned to was the Paleo diet—a diet consisting chiefly of lean meats, seafood, fruits, vegetables, nuts and seeds and health fats, and excluding dairy, grain products, legumes, starches, and processed food. It's a popular for inflammatory and autoimmune issues, among others. This diet is rich in alkaline and anti-inflammatory foods, so it arms the body with its best defenses, helping it to stay diseases-free for a long, healthy life. With this diet, one can proposedly lose fat and stay young while avoiding cancer, diabetes, heart disease, Parkinson's, Alzheimer's disease, and other illnesses.

Some components of the Paleo diet are increased protein and reduced carbohydrate intake, higher fiber intake, higher potassium and lower sodium intake, and higher vitamin, mineral, and antioxidant intake. For a good online resource, go to thepaleodiet. com, there you can learn more about the diet and access recipes. Also, Robb Wolf, author of the *New York Times* bestseller *The Paleo Solution*, offers a way to get started quickly and some great information at robbwolf.com.

Benefits of a Health Coach

If you are looking for that inspiration or motivation to help you elevate your health and overall lifestyle, you might be looking for a health coach. While food is one area of interest, health coaches offer help with vast issues with the goal of balancing important elements of your life such as love and relationships as well as career and money.

A health coach will personally guide you to make simple, small ongoing changes that ultimately transform your life. Health coaches inspire individuals to realize the value in reaching their health-related goals and building a meaningful connection between exercise and activities of daily living. Once a person understands this value, they are empowered to create positive, lasting lifestyle changes that enhance what they do in the gym, outdoors, on the way to work, and in any facet of their everyday life.

Instead of treating the symptoms, health coaches will work with their clients to get to the underlying cause of their health concerns. We look at how issues such as stress, emotional distress, physical activities, lack of soul nourishment and other personal factors affect each individual's overall well-being. Helping cultivate an awareness arms clients with information for a lifetime.

As a passionate advocate of the ripple effect, health coaches are truly changing the way people live; the more of us that are out there doing this work, the greater the change will be. As a result, we are having a tremendous influence on the world's health.

You can learn more about health coaching on my website: www. simplifyhealthfitness.com.

Eating Clean—What Does It Mean?

Eating clean is an often-heard term these days. It is the practice of avoiding processed and refined foods in favor of whole foods. Whole foods haven't been tampered with in the lab or the manufacturing plant. They are straight from the farm: whole fruits and vegetables, whole grains, grass-fed and free-range meats, low fat dairy products, unsalted nuts, and seeds.

Processed foods are almost any food that has a label. A label means that more than one ingredient was used to make that food. (There are some exceptions, like whole grain pasta and natural cheeses.)

Tips for the Produce Aisle

If you are considering an organic diet, the labeling on produce can help. Produce with a five-digit PLU code (price lookup number) starting with a nine is organic. Five-digit numbers starting with an eight are GMOs (genetically modified organisms) and should be avoided. A four-digit number indicates grown by conventional means.

Sometimes moving from conventional to organic produce is not the most important consideration. According to the Environmental Working Group, by avoiding the most contaminated produce consumers can reduce exposure to pesticides by 80 percent. This list is referred to as the Dirty Dozen. You can save some money and find peace of mind by choosing conventional produce from the Clean 15 list: the produce found to have the lowest pesticide content.

DIRTY DOZEN	CLEAN 15
Highest pesticide Content	*Lowest pesticide Content*
Apples	Avocados
Peaches	Sweet Corn
Nectarines	Pineapples
Strawberries	Cabbage
Grapes	Sweet Peas (frozen)
Celery	Onions
Spinach	Asparagus
Sweet Bell Peppers	Mangoes
Cucumbers	Papayas
Cherry Tomatoes	Kiwi
Snap Peas (Imported)	Eggplant
Potatoes	Grapefruit
	Cantaloupe
	Cauliflower
	Sweet Potatoes

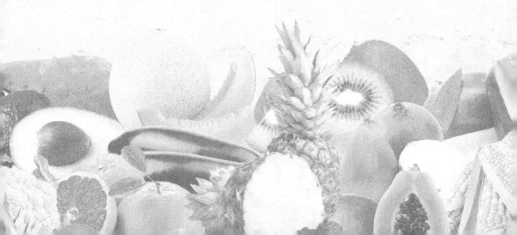

What Is Vinyasa Yoga?

Stretch, flex and find your center

The word *vinyasa* can be translated as "arranging something in a special way." Vinyasa yoga is based on postures and breathing techniques. Its beauty comes from sequential interlinking postures leading to a continuous flow. Vinyasa yoga offers many health benefits, from stretching aching muscles to finding inner peace and much more.

Yoga at a Glance

Yoga can improve flexibility, concentration, and performance. It is widely known to reduce stress, deliver a sense of inner peace, and renew self-confidence. With regular practice, yoga can lead to an advanced state, creating a deep, harmonious connection to spirit, and a sense of oneness between body, mind, spirit, and the Universe.

This ancient stretching and strength discipline may look pretty, but it also benefits the big guys. Many athletes from pro football to baseball and even rugby have incorporated yoga. Men's Fitness reports that some pro football teams, such as the New York Giants and Philadelphia Eagles, have added yoga into their rigorous training routines. Also, many major sports teams and athletes work yoga into their pre- and off-season workouts. Most pro football teams have a few players practicing yoga regularly. If that weren't enough, the New

Zealand All Blacks rugby team hit a rough patch leading to rocky performance. The club hired a yoga instructor for some help, according to MSN. The team reportedly benefited from the visualization techniques saying they were a good preparation tool for upcoming games.

How Yoga Helped Me

I never gave yoga much credence but turned to it as a practice for healing. Then I started experiencing lasting results. Yoga helped me with balance, inner peace, and bolstered energy. Yoga is not only a physical practice; it serves practitioners mentally, emotionally, and spiritually too, which is why everyone from corporate leaders to football players are turning to it for that extra edge.

My regard for yoga grew so much that I ultimately completed a comprehensive two-hundred-hour yoga teacher training in Vinyasa yoga, and I became registered with the Yoga Alliance as a RYT200 yoga instructor. This achievement was a wonderful gift for my mind, body, and soul.

The Benefits of Yoga

- Inspire balance
- Release fear
- Restore calm
- Heal gracefully
- Empower transformation
- Embrace joy
- Achieve goals
- Improve focus
- Improve circulation

- Improve balance
- Eases fibromyalgia conditions related to joint and muscle pain

Ocean Breath—Ujjayi Pranayama Breathing

Ujjayi Pranayama is one of the most powerful breaths and is wonderful to do during the physical practice of yoga as it energizes the body and centers the mind. This method will help bring oxygen into your system while creating a calm, focused state of mind. In translation, *ujjayi* means victorious and *pranayama* means to stretch or extend the prana, or life force.

Ocean breath is not a translation of Ujjayi breath (victorious breath); instead it reflects the sound the breath creates, reminiscent of the sound a wave makes rolling up and back down a beach. It is achieved by controlling the movement of breath into and back out of the body.

Ujjayi Prep

Sit in sukhasana ("easy pose," with legs crossed). Roll up a towel to place against the base of your spine to support your posture or find the best way to support your seated position.

At first, breathe normally and observe what you can about what your breath indicates regarding your body and mind. Is it rapid, slow, uneven, maybe shallow?

We can influence our mind and body through our breath. Likewise, our breath tells us a great deal about what is happening within our body.

Steady your breath by counting to five as you inhale; then count to five as you exhale.

Ujjayi Pranayama

1. Sit in a sukhasana ("easy pose," with legs crossed). Use props such as a rolled towel just under your spine to maintain comfort while lengthening your spine. Drop your shoulders and keep your chin parallel to floor.
2. Rest your hands on your knees and close your eyes.
3. Inhale to a count of five. Open your mouth. As you exhale, contract your throat and make an "hhhaaa" sound, as if you were fogging a mirror.
4. Now close your mouth and breathe through your nose only, but continue making this "hhhaaa" sound with each inhale and exhale. As your breath moves through your contracted throat, it makes the sound of ocean waves. Doing this during yoga increases your sense of reach, stretch and strength. Victorious!

This is the ujjayi pranayama breathing method. Next time you are practicing yoga, try employing it on long stretches. It makes the experience more beneficial because you will bring oxygen to your body at a time that you are working major muscles. Until then, continue the practice as above.

The Almighty Sun

Illuminate your day with sun salutations

Over centuries and across cultures, two things have stayed the same: the sun and the value so many people have placed on light as a symbol of good and self-illumination. The sun has long been worshiped as a great sign of light. Hindus called the sun "surya" and viewed it as the physical and spiritual heart of our world and creator of all life.

The sun salutation sequence practiced in multiple styles of yoga is a series of asanas designed to warm up the body and open the mind and heart before starting further yoga practice or simply to be done in repetition on its own. The name "sun salutation" in Sanskrit is "surya" (sun), "namaskar," which stems from *namas*, meaning "to bow to" or "to adore." In the familiar yoga term *namaste, te* means "you."

The series of postures work the entire body—stretching, flexing, and toning major and minor muscles through the core, arms, shoulders, calves, thighs, and hips. This a great way to get the "yoga butt" that everyone talks about. Physical and emotional balance is improved, and many health benefits beyond the physical level can be achieved, such as mental relaxation leading into meditation.

The sun salutation is a beautiful way to show gratitude to the sun and to your inner spirit. Each time you flow through this sequence, you will synchronize your breath with the movement of your body; for example, sweeping your arms open wide and up, taking in a great breath, then swooping down, exhaling with intent, always breathing through the nose, not the mouth. Focus on the inhale or exhale through your movements, always beginning and ending with joined hands, mudra (gesture), touched to the heart. Only the heart can know the truth.

SURYA NAMASKAR A

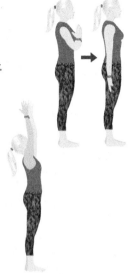

1 **TADASANA** (Mountain Pose)
- Stand tall to the front edge of your mat with your feet hip width and heels 2 inches apart. Connect your hands to your heart center.
- Gaze forward, distribute your weight evenly over both feet.
- Establish a slow, steady rhythm for your breath.
- **EXHALE**, to bring your arms down by your side.

2 **URDVA HASTASANA** (Upward salute)
- **INHALE**, reach your arms up toward the sky and join your palms.
- Raise your gaze to your hands and slide your shoulders away from your ears and your shoulder blades down your back.
- Engage your legs and lift up through the arches of the feet.

3 **UTTANSANA** (Standing Forward Bend)
- **EXHALE**, fold forward from the waist, bringing your arms down and placing your hands to the earth, or you can place them on your shins or a block.
- Relax the back of your neck and shift some weight into the balls of your feet.

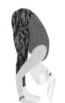

4 **ARDHA UTTANSANA** (Half Forward Bend)
- **INHALE**, as you lift your torso halfway, lengthening your spine forward so your back is flat.
- The gaze is lifted, the spine is extended, and the fingertips can stay on the floor or rise to the shins.

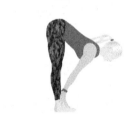

5 **CHATURANGA DANDASANA** (Four Limb Staff Pose)
- **EXHALE**, as you step back into Plank position, with your hands under your shoulders and feet hip distance apart.
- Continue exhaling as you lower your body toward the floor.
- Keep your elbows tucked in toward your sides.
- Your shoulders should align with the elbows and elbows should align with the wrists.

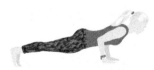

6 **ASHTANGA NAMASKARA** (Knee, chest, chin)
- Lower your body down till your knees, chest and chin are touching the mat, and the hip and abdomen is slightly raised up.

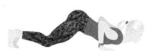

SURYA NAMASKAR A cont'd

7 **BHUJANGASANA** (Cobra)

- **INHALE**, slide your body forward, lift your chest while keeping your elbows bent, close to the ribs, thighs and hips remain contact with the floor, eyes follow the tip of the nose.

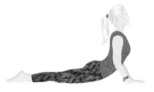

8 **ADHO MUKHA SVANASANA** (Downward Facing Dog)

- **EXHALE**, push to a plank, lift your hips placing the soles of your feet on the earth.
- Stack your shoulders directly above your wrists and hips directly above your knees.
- Ground down through your hands and the soles of your feet as you lengthen your spine.
- Lift your belly and sit bones toward the sky.
- Stretch your heels down towards the mat.

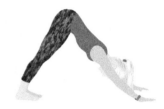

9 **ARDHA UTTANSANA** (Half Forward Bend)

- **INHALE**, walk or jump your the feet to the front of the mat raising to lengthen the spine, gazing slightly forward.

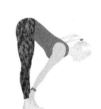

10 **UTTANSANA** (Standing Forward Bend)

- **EXHALE**, fold forward and try to bring your head as close as possible to your knees.

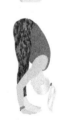

11 **TADASANA** (Mountain Pose)

- **INHALE**, bringing your hands to heart center.

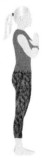

SURYA NAMASKAR B

1 TADASANA (Mountain Pose)

- Connect your hands to your heart center firmly. Ground your feet to the mat and feel the crown of your head drawing upward toward the sky.
- **EXHALE**, to bring your arms down by your side.

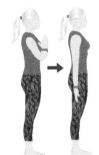

2 UTKATASANA (Chair Pose)

- **INHALE**, standing with your big toes touching, your heels slightly apart, bend your knees, and lower your hips, extend your arms straight overhead and reach through your fingertips.

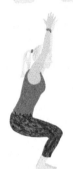

3 UTTANSANA (Standing Forward Bend)

- **EXHALE**, fold forward letting your body melt down toward the earth.
- If your hands don't reach the floor, bend your knees slightly.

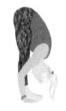

4 ARDHA UTTANSANA (Half Forward Bend)

- **INHALE**, to lengthen the spine coming into a flat back.
- The gaze is slightly forward.
- Activate your thighs to lift out of your kneecaps.

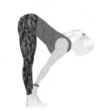

5 CHATURANGA DANDASANA (Four Limb Staff Pose)

- **EXHALE**, as you step back into Plank position, with your hands under your shoulders and feet hip distance apart.
- Continue exhaling as you lower your body toward the floor.
- Keep your elbows tucked in toward your sides.
- Your shoulders should align with the elbows and elbows should align with the wrists.

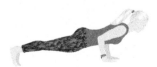

SURYA NAMASKAR B cont'd

⑥ URDHVA MUKHA SVANASANA (Upward Facing Dog)

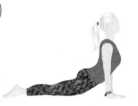

- **INHALE**, legs extended behind you.
- Press the balls of the feet toward the back of the mat.
- Place your hands on the floor alongside your body, next to your lower ribs.
- Point your fingers to the top of the mat and hug your elbows in dose to your ribcage.
- Broaden through the collarbones, lift from the heart and feel the shoulders sliding down the back.

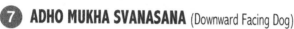

⑦ ADHO MUKHA SVANASANA (Downward Facing Dog)

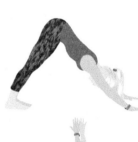

- **EXHALE**, push to a plank, lift your hips placing the soles of your feet on the earth.
- Align your wrists directly under your shoulders and your knees directly under your hips.
- Stretch your heels down towards the mat.

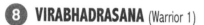

⑧ VIRABHADRASANA (Warrior 1)

- **INHALE**, step the **LEFT FOOT** forward and pivot inwards at a 45 degree angle, align your front heel with the arch of your back foot.
- Keep your pelvis turned toward the front of your mat.
- Reach up strongly through your arms, keep your palms and fingers active and reaching.
- Drop the shoulders from the ears.

⑨ CHATURANGA DANDASANA (Four Limb Staff Pose)

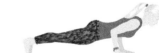

- **EXHALE**, cartwheel your hands to the front of the mat into a plank, lower your body toward the floor.

⑩ URDHVA MUKHA SVANASANA (Upward Facing Dog)

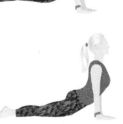

- **INHALE**, hands directly under shoulders, chest lifts; hips and knees are off the floor.
- Weight is on the top of your toes.

SURYA NAMASKAR B cont'd

⑪ ADHO MUKHA SVANASANA (Downward Facing Dog)

- **EXHALE**, rotate the inner thighs back, ground down through your hands and the soles of your feet as you lengthen your spine.
- Soften the neck and draw the heels towards the mat.

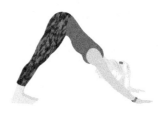

⑫ VIRABHADRASANA (Right Foot Warrior 1)

- **INHALE**, step the **RIGHT FOOT** forward and pivot inwards at a 45 degree angle, align your front heel with the arch of your back foot.
- Keep your pelvis turned toward the front of your mat.
- Reach up strongly through your arms, keep your palms and fingers active and reaching.
- Drop the shoulders from the ears.

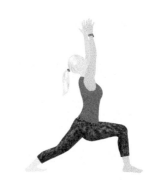

⑬ CHATURANGA DANDASANA (Four Limb Staff Pose)

- **INHALE**, walk or jump your the feet to the front of the mat raising to lengthen the spine, gazing slightly forward.

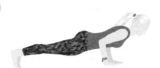

⑭ URDHVA MUKHA SVANASANA (Upward Facing Dog)

- **INHALE**, press the balls of the feet toward the back of the mat. Place your hands on the floor alongside your body, next to your lower ribs.

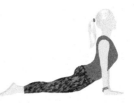

⑮ ADHO MUKHA SVANASANA (Downward Facing Dog)

- **EXHALE**, rotate the inner thighs back ground down through your hands and the soles of your feet as you lengthen your spine.
- Soften the neck and draw the heels towards the mat.

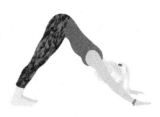

SURYA NAMASKAR B cont'd

16 ARDHA UTTANSANA (Half Forward Bend)

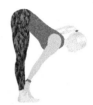

* **INHALE**, walk or jump your the feet to the front of the mat raising to lengthen the spine, gazing slightly forward.

17 UTTANSANA (Standing Forward Bend)

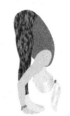

* **EXHALE**, fold forward from the waist, bringing your arms down and placing your hands to the earth, or you can place them on your shins or a block.

18 UTKATASANA (Chair Pose)

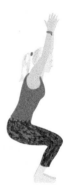

* **INHALE**, bend your knees, and lower your hips, extend your arms straight overhead and reach through your fingertips.

19 TADASANA (Mountain Pose)

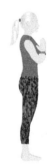

* **EXHALE**, bringing your hands to heart center.

Ayurveda
The newest solutions are the oldest

Ayurveda is a practice that spans thousands of years and many countries. Those who practice Ayurveda reportedly can live more than one hundred years, with this data reaching back as far as the practice itself. If you want to feel healthy, vibrant, full of energy, and at ease, Ayurveda is a practice treating all human conditions and might be right for you.

Ayurveda is treatment-specific to each person. Therapy is intended to bring ease into a person's life and support all levels of their unique mind and body's health, daily activities, and self-care routines.

It is an extremely broad practice primarily focusing on living a life of balance. Your practitioner would assess you, then guide you through the development of an exclusive plan that comfortably fits your needs:

- Diet, lifestyle, and herbal solutions for a wide variety of issues from anxiety to digestion and more
- Aromatherapy, skincare, and practicing gratitude
- A focus on perfect health mentally and physically
- Seasonal routines and night routines
- Ayurveda also taps into sound therapy, the chakras, breath awareness, gem therapy, nadis, meditation, and yoga if any are appropriate

If you would like to learn more about ayurveda, opportunities to attend workshops, read up, or get certified are growing more popular and accessible. A little online research should help you find some nearby activities; if not, perhaps you and some friends can form a study group. You might become the first to start an ayurveda group in your area. If you do, drop me an e-mail! My website is on the back of this book.

On the medical side, ayurveda is an integrative, noninvasive medical practice. A BAMS (bachelor of ayurvedic medicine and surgery) is a graduate degree requiring five and a half years' study, including a one-year internship. The curriculum includes modern anatomy, forensic medicine, physiology, pharmacology, toxicology, ear-nose-throat, ophthalmology, preventive and social medicine, principles of surgery, and more, plus ayurvedic topics.

Ayurvedic health counselors are on the rise. The health counselor evaluates a patient's constitution and any imbalance, then focuses on disease prevention by devising proper dietary and lifestyle changes. They use herbal formulas to balance the digestive system, mind, emotions, and other areas that might require balancing or healing at times.

Ayurvedic practitioners are becoming more popular in the United States. The practice treats each patient based on their unique constitution and combination of life forces, known as *doshas* (see next section), which determine the patient's physical and psychological health and vulnerabilities. Using certain noninvasive tests, an ayurvedic practitioner creates a regimen for the patient to balance their wellness.

- As of 2010, 40 percent of adults were using complementary or alternative medicine.
- Ayurveda is a popular study for massage therapists, others offering services at a wellness center or give yoga lessons or are simply living a life based on yoga practices.
- Yoga and ayurveda are sister sciences and have similarities.

The Doshas
Maximize your energy right now

The Five Elements

The ancient Indian term *ayurveda* means "science of life." The practice of ayurvedic medicine is based on an understanding that our bodies, like the environment, are comprised of five elements: *air, space, fire, water, and earth*. Health is viewed as the state of balance between mind, body, and environment, along with the soul.

Our balance with the environment is clearly important. We must be in balance to be able to breathe in our environment (not everyone can; thus some of us are not in balance, and health *can* be viewed this way), and eat the meat and vegetables from our environment. We cannot survive without proper hydration, and neither can our food, be it animal or vegetable, so water is crucial. We also need fire for more things than any of us can count, from cooking to crop control, to sanitizing for just a few examples.

Of course we each balance with our environment in our own way. Along with our ability to breathe with ease, consider such physical or emotional effects as allergies, arthritis, bursitis, migraines, and seasonal affect disorder. This is the individuality in our relationship with the environment and a simple illustration for why an individual assessment and treatment is the basis of all ayurvedic care.

The mind-body balance is just as important. Most anything we do physically is impacted emotionally: a peaceful walk, a long, rough day, preparing food, and cleaning, for a few examples. Any mental experience affects us physically: a major win, loss, falling in love, breaking up, a discovery or victory, and so on. Our adrenal glands work hard, endorphins are released, our posture changes, and so does our appetite and effort to sleep for a few examples.

Uncovering the Doshas

In ayurveda, the five elements (air, space, fire, water, and earth) are applied such that any two combine to express a specific energy type. A person's physical and physiological makeup is defined by that combination of two elements. There are three possible outcomes; ayurveda calls these *doshas*. The energies (e.g., fire and water) circulate throughout the mind-body and govern physiological activity.

The doshas represent our dominant selves. This easy-to-garner information helps tailor a personal diet and lifestyle for optimum health, a general sense of ease, and mental and emotional peace.

Quick tests are available that uncover your dominant dosha, such as this one, from deepak chopra:

http://doshaquiz.chopra.com/

If you took the test, you determined that you are a vata, a pitta, or a kapha. Each of these doshas contain two of the five elements:

- **Vata:** a combination of air and space.
- **Pitta:** a combination of fire and water.
- **Kapha:** a combination of earth and water.

Your Self-Assessment

Next, each of the three doshas are described with some tips to keep you feeling well and balanced mentally, physically, and spiritually.

Vata Type – *Thin, light, enthusiastic, energetic, and changeable*
Predominant vata doshas are very active and energetic. Always on the go, they battle with restlessness. They forget as quickly as they learn. Having fast metabolisms, they are generally thin and might wrestle with a sensitive digestion. Vatas love excitement and new experiences. They are lively, joyous, and creative. They are so enthusiastic and have high energy that their sleep is light.

When out of balance, Vatas are more likely to suffer insomnia, anxiety, headaches, difficulty focusing, dry skin, sore throats, abdominal gas, constipation, and neurological disorders. This is likely due to their high-energy, fast-moving lifestyle.

To balance vata: maintain a flexible body and daily routine.

- Bring warmth, stability, and consistency to your life. Try to get to bed before 10:00 p.m. and awaken by 6:00 a.m. Also eat meals on a regular schedule.
- Use fresh ginger root frequently.
- Routine massage treatments help to release tight muscles and sooth the mind and body, reducing that high-frequency energy.
- Choose light exercise options that enhance balance and flexibility like yoga, taichi, short hikes, or golf.

Pitta Type – *Intense, intellectual, and goal-oriented*

Pitta-type people are usually strong, of medium size, and well-built. Pittas are warm, friendly, organized, and bright. They possess strong management skills, discipline, and ambition. Pittas' flair as public speakers make them natural leaders. Their sexual vigor is greater than vatas but less than kaphas. Pittas enjoy spending money and lavish assets. Pittas do not do well with too much sunlight or intense heat.

Out-of-balance Pittas can face inner or outer surface area disease. Their love for being the leader, a show runner, and in the public can become a strain. Pittas risk compulsive and irritable behavior. Their skin may suffer from hypersensitivity, rashes, hives and dry patches, or acne. Other pitta issues include heartburn and ulcers, inflammatory issues, thinning hair, indigestion, and high blood pressure.

To balance pitta: *aim for calm and solitude*

- Choose activities or relaxation that steadies or calms and cools.
- Take some free time for journaling, free writing, or a simple rest to recharge your body daily.
- Spend time in nature regularly. This is a great way to get connected with your true self.
- Use sparingly hotter spices like ginger, cumin, fenugreek, black pepper, clove, salt, and mustard seed. Avoid very hot seasonings like chili peppers and cayenne.
- Meditate regularly. It can help ease the mind, release issues of control, and dissipate anger.

  Other calming activities include swimming, walking in nature, and gardening.

Kapha Type – *Easygoing, methodical, and nurturing*

Kapha types are resilient, stable, and calm. They tend to have a strong, large build and high muscle development. Kaphas tend to be thoughtful, supportive, and loving. They like to prepare and enjoy gourmet foods. They might take their time learning, but they have exceptional memories. Kaphas tend to have a slow, steady pace. They enjoy long, deep sleep.

If kapha is out of balance, they might sleep too much, feel sluggish, experience weight gain, and risk sinus congestion, water retention, depression, asthma, diabetes, cysts, edema, or swelling.

To balance kapha: *spice it up and get moving*

- Enjoy light, dry, and warm foods.
- Use heating spices such as chili, black, or cayenne pepper, cinnamon, ginger, and cumin. These ingredients can stimulate a slow metabolism.
- Reduce all nuts.
- Avoid highly processed foods, cold or carbonated drinks, red meat, and alcohol. Processed foods contain chemicals that increase edema, water retention, and a sense of bliss from processed ingredients, which cause overeating and a false need to eat again sooner.
- A vital, hearty exercise routine of jogging, hiking, biking, vigorous forms of yoga or martial arts or other challenging forms of exercise, at least five times per week. Try many things until a few click. Ayurveda aligns treatment with lifestyle and choices. You should feel joy,, and it is acceptable to mix it up to achieve a five times per week goal. Bring a friend; make it fun.

SOUL

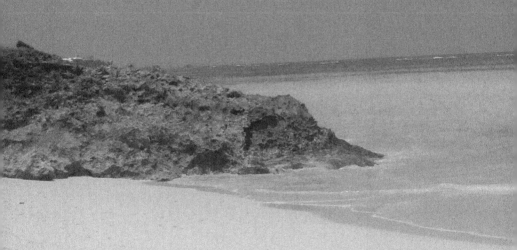

Put your heart, mind, and soul into even
your smallest acts. This is the secret to success.
- Swami Sivananda -

Spirituality

Understand this, understand everything

Birth

We are born into this earthly existence a spiritual being. Before we begin on our life on earth, we are souls. We arrive spiritual. We forget as we are bombarded with earth life, right from the first spank. In fact, the first cue that earth will be a hard place filled with tests and challenges is the actual experience of being born. Birth is the hardest thing we ever do. Our naturally curious human brain is immediately hungry to learn and capable of complex thought. Our mental, physical, physiological, and emotional makeup along with the characteristics of life on earth makes forgetting our spiritual selves a natural, albeit unfortunate, outcome. It's important to start by remembering this truth: we are spiritual beings in earthly bodies trying to exist in an earthly world, not the other way around.

Let Go

The key is to understand that we don't have a playbook for life. We don't have the power to control outcomes, and we certainly do not know if an outcome is good or bad because we cannot see the future and how this outcome affects it. Are you grateful for a red light? Thankful you didn't get the job? What would have happened next if the light had been green? Do you know?

Once the barriers most of us seem to adopt and learn are released, forgiven, and freed, we are better able to watch for the upcoming good when faced with such things as not getting a certain job, a relationship coming to its endpoint, or even the death of a loved one. Have you noticed that the folks who react with a smile, even in the roughest situations, seem to be graced with the next amazing opportunity quickly? Contrast that with those who wallow in sadness: they never go anywhere soon, if ever. They are weighed down and, moreover, shut down, which makes it impossible for them to be grateful or see any reason to use their past experience for good. Faced with this fate, opportunity cannot be blessed. The more we learn to doubt, fear, and "protect ourselves," the less we live our spiritual greatness, instead faced with life in this limited earthly existence. Had I shut down forever instead of fighting when I lost my mother, I would not have this opportunity to tell this story today.

Moreover, the degree to which we try to write another human being's story, presuming we know better than our Creator what this other person is meant to experience, learn, face in life, or become is foolish when we stand back and realize what we are doing. What educational focus they want or any real choices they make should be left to flourish in most instances and within obvious reason. Certainly you are acting out of love or basing your actions on your own experience and "knowing better," but we are not here to keep everyone from sidestepping our education and developing the muscles, courage, and proper background to someday become what they were put here to be.

None of us know what each other's purpose is; not even a mother knows her own child's life purpose, as difficult as that may be. Letting go will bring you peace, and the more you let go, the more you will gain in terms of balance, insight, and good fortune in your life. As you let go more and more, your spiritual self will become primary in your life.

The most important thing you will learn if you do let go, stop worrying, just be in the moment, and trust that all is well, is that there wasn't anything to hold on to in the first place. It is all false, earth-based ideas that are unrealistic. Open your clenched hand and see it is empty. Open your mind in meditation. Let go… really let go, and discover how far you can see when excessive worry, fear, or attempts to control the unknown are out of your way. Open your body slowly, through yoga and qigong; see how free you can feel, how pain drifts away when you stop carrying the weight of this temporary place or someone else's story, which you will never fully understand, on your shoulders. All of this is spiritual and natural to you.

The Spiritual Lens and Connecting

When you see life through a spiritual lens, you see possibility where you once saw limitation. Outcomes aren't bad; they're just outcomes, and you know that they happen to make way for the next step, the next blessing, the next amazing part of life.

Many of us discover this during meditation, yoga, or qigong, attending mass, during Shabbat, or on consistent long walks through nature. Journaling also helps because that which holds us captive, such as anger, resentment, worry, or fear, can be put onto paper where now *we* own *it*. It is amazing how the power balance swings once an issue is put to paper. Sometimes as we write, we surprise ourselves at what comes onto the paper. Uncovering what's really eating us is the first step to getting a handle on it.

A journal also helps us to look back and see the level at which we attached ourselves to other peoples' behaviors or judgments; sometimes this means others' addictions or other abusive behaviors. Hopefully we come to understand that we are all on a level playing field; none of us are higher or lower than the other; some are at one stage and others at another in their life, however; and if you think you can resolve another person's challenges, you might be cutting them short in their journey of learning and becoming prepared for something they are slated to achieve. Is that your call? If you have a level of ability to help and that is your role, then great! Follow your instincts; when that help is done, we all must know to let go.

Letting go is so key to spirituality because it reflects true nature of being. No spiritual being is in charge of another spiritual being. Also, any attachment to another person or any event in life must be released for a person to evolve. There is no attaining your greatest potentiality while holding on tightly to something that by the nature of attachment thus holds some of your personal power. Remember, this other individual has their own book; you cannot change their story. When they find their answers, they are blessed with amazing calling that might have nothing to do with yours. You certainly can share this information with them, perhaps inspiring personal change.

Be Grateful and See Things in a Positive Way

One way to understand spirituality is through a "spiritual glasses" analogy. This is something you can apply any time you face a confusing or difficult situation or simply in daily life. The spiritual glasses offer a view that helps you see the situation in a more open, positive, enlightened way. They make it easy to be grateful and help you get ready for something wonderful and new at all times but especially when things might otherwise take away your power, shut you down, and zap your energy.

Imagine you are sitting across the desk from your boss who is working through the difficult task of letting you go. You can struggle, negotiate, fight, analyze the situation, place blame, and get depressed, or you can put on those spiritual glasses. Through the glasses, you see a beautiful being, maybe an angel, right next to your boss. (Please note that I am giving you an image only as a way of producing the idea of how you would view the situation and not intending you will begin actually seeing angels.) This image is all in white and smiling at you knowingly as they open a big ornate door. As you watch this moment unfold, your spiritual self realizes if you don't get out of this mundane life that revolves around this job, you won't be ready for the better thing coming your way.

Did you really think you would do that job, retire, then sit at home sipping coffee and reading newspapers and that would be it? This is your spiritual side. Your ever-alert wake-up call saying, "There's more to you. There are so many blessings for you if you rise up and accept them." Your spiritual glasses are there for you in any situation; they will guide your light and happy, grateful self to see things in a positive way.

Intent, Gratitude, and Belief in the Best

Living a spiritual life means living with intent, gratitude, and belief in the best. If you have driven a car at night, you know that your headlights only show you a few feet ahead, yet you are relaxed and filled with faith that your path will end in success. You know without proof that at the end of your drive you will get out of your car and be where you intend to be. The intent with which we travel in the night is no different than the intent with which our spiritual selves operate. If you are relaxed and filled with faith that your path will end in success, it will. What you intend will be.

The best fuel for a spiritual existence is gratitude. A grateful person is happy and satisfied. "Gratitude brings on the best attitude," they say. Further, if you are grateful, you are prepared to accept more. One of the best ways to end or begin each day is with a few minutes of gratitude. Think about your many blessings and be grateful for them.

Forgiveness

Let go and get your power back

Possibly the biggest roadblock to growth and transformation is an inability to forgive. Lack of forgiveness has kept family, friends, neighbors, business associates, and countries apart for centuries. One of the greatest reasons we are so stubborn to let the other guy off the hook is that we don't realize who benefits from doing so.

The truth is there is nothing so powerful as letting go. Letting go of old clothes, excess files, collections you really never liked and always had to dust, and resentment or anger. Letting go is so freeing it literally feels like cool fresh air engulfing you as weights lift from your tired shoulders. Suddenly your mind clears as though your brain has freed up space for new and much more stimulating thought. When you forgive someone, you let go. It does nothing for them. They don't even have to know about it; it does a world of good for you.

So long as you continue to hold a grudge, that other person has some of your personal power. Some portion of your energy rests with them until you take it back. Whether you know it or not, while you remain in a relationship of this nature, you deposit your energy into that person's hands. Moreover, when we are legitimately upset with somebody our ability to receive guidance from a greater source is blocked. Anger, bitter thoughts, anything that stops us from forgiving also blocks us from achieving, and we achieve like gangbusters when we are open to greater guidance. These two power centers—personal power and greater guidance can be bolstered simply by forgiving.

To forgive does not mean you accept what happened. The word *forgive* has a feel and a vibe to it that makes it difficult to work with. *Forgive* sounds like, "I have decided it is okay with me. I am no longer uncomfortable or upset." This is not forgiveness. Think of forgiveness as a giant scissors and the problem, issue, behavior, or relationship as a big rope. You and this individual are tethered together by the rope. As you attempt to move forward with your life, you must haul this person along with you. They define you in certain ways because they were part of a time gone by, so you are unable to let go of many things that are connected to that person. Wherever you go, you must haul this weight with you. You can't update your ways entirely; maybe you are stuck with an outdated wardrobe or keep saying it's time for a complete hair makeover, but it's all talk, and you cannot figure out why. It's that rope. You are holding yourself back. The most interesting thing about two people holding a grudge is standing back and observing them—not the grudge, but all the other things about them and their lives. All the limitations they would lose if they cut that rope, and they have no idea they are only hurting themselves, often in some big ways.

You don't have to like the past, and maybe today or in a year or someday you will learn from it. Right now, slicing that rope makes you free, light, and ready to go. You give it a cosmic slice, and off you go to the opportunities that await. You notice after cutting the line that you don't miss it. You no longer feel like talking about it. You feel excited as a sudden rush of new ideas floods your cleared mind. Your sights are on today and your bright tomorrow, and your personal power swells.

This is forgiveness. It is letting go. It is about reducing the anger and resentment in the world. The payoff for each forgiveness is huge; you always move forward and benefit more than you'll know when you let go of something hurtful, wrong, or in any way negative from the past.

Forgiveness is hard until you get the hang of it. At first, it won't feel sincere or natural. As delicious as the outcomes are, this is a deep-seated emotional issue that you have carried for a while; how can you just cut a pretend rope and evolve? The key here is to step back from your side of the issue and evaluate the other person. Whatever they did, something led them to that behavior. Maybe they are emotionally weaker or unable to determine right from wrong. Could they be jealous of you? Perhaps there is something about their family background that aided in creating this glitch in their behavior. They might even be acting out at you based on bad information, and you might have to swallow that pill and let them go on with their life thinking they were right. Knowing the why behind their action sometimes helps with the good-bye.

Sometimes you don't have access to any information, and you just have to cut that rope and do it again and again until you come to discover the truth: You are not this person's god or coach. You cannot control them or change them. You will never be able to go back in time, so there is no reason to hold on when you are holding on to absolutely nothing. When you cut them loose they, and the situation, will be gone and done. One day soon you will cut them loose, and this time, it will be final. No phone number in the cell, all done and freedom at last. Any reminder or proof you have been keeping goes out with the trash.

You will come to realize that the other person is serving a purpose in your life. When that "aha" moment comes, you will want to thank your nemesis for tripping you up. This is the best kind of forgiveness, the enlightened forgiveness. Don't wait for everything to be crystal clear to forgive. Someday all will come to light. For now, grow into forgiveness by forgiving and evolving. Truth be told, this was all set ahead of time and part of a path you had to take, so take it. Moving forward is much more fun, and feels so good.

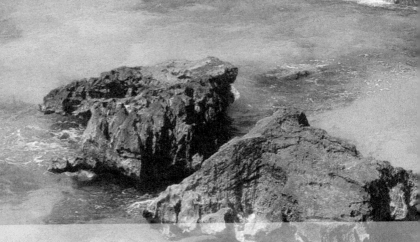

INSPIRING
AWARENESS
FAST

Be the change you wish to see in the World.
- Ghandi -

Understanding Stroke

Save a life, maybe your own

If you experience stroke symptoms or witness a stroke in progress, the information in this section will empower you with simple but necessary life-saving action steps. You will also learn what is true and what the myths are surrounding this highly preventable disease. Also, the types of strokes will be discussed. Each type of stroke comes with different risks and outcomes.

Misconceptions

Stroke is a longstanding disease, yet most have at least one or two misconceptions about it. Many think that stroke only happens to the elderly when in fact it can occur anytime to anyone including children. Eighty percent of strokes can be prevented, and while some believe it cannot be treated, the truth is that the faster a person gets treatment, the better their chances are for a full recovery. Those individuals who do receive emergency treatment will continue to recover over the span of the rest of their lives. The brain continually undergoes repair, and there is no timeframe within which stroke recovery is limited. Also, stroke is sometimes called a brain attack, to clarify and separate it from the heart, which would, of course, have a heart attack.

To understand more about preventing stroke, it is important to bring up questions regarding stroke with your physician. Stroke is the fifth cause of death and a leading cause of serious, long-term disability in America. Each year, 795,000 Americans will have a stroke and 160,000 people will die as a result, according to the National Stroke Association.

The Basics

- Check the time so you know when the first symptoms appeared.
- Recognize the stroke warning signs. People may experience some or all the signs.
- Even if the warning signs go away, continue treating the situation as life-threatening.

Stroke Warning Signs

People may experience some or all of these signs:

- Sudden numbness or weakness of the face, arm, or leg, mainly on one side of the body.
- Sudden confusion, trouble speaking, or understanding.
- Sudden trouble seeing in one or both eyes.
- Sudden trouble walking, dizziness, loss of balance, or coordination.
- Sudden severe headache with no known cause.

FAST is an easy way to remember how to recognize a stroke and what to do:

- **F**ace drooping – Does one side of the face droop, or is it numb?
- **A**rm weakness – Is one arm weak or numb?
- **S**peech difficulty – Is speech slurred?
- **T**ime to call 9-1-1 – Get the person to the hospital immediately.

Details about Stroke

There are two primary types of stroke, hemorrhagic and ischemic. Only 15 percent of strokes are hemorrhagic, but they account for about 40 percent of all stroke-related deaths.

Hemorrhagic strokes can be intracerebral (within the brain) or subarachnoid (surrounding the brain). These happen from a blood vessel that ruptures and bleeds or a brain aneurism burst.

Intracerebral Hemorrhage

An intracerebral hemorrhage happens when blood suddenly bursts into brain tissue, causing damage to the brain. Signs include headache, confusion, weakness, and paralysis, mainly on one side of the body. Blood buildup puts pressure on the brain, interfering with oxygen supply and risking brain and nerve damage.

Subarachnoid Hemorrhage

Subarachnoid hemorrhages cause bleeding between the brain and the tissues that cover it, risking coma, paralysis, and even death. This type of hemorrhage comes on fast. The primary sign is a sudden severe headache that is more intense at the base of the skull. Seek immediate medical help if the person experiences this headache along with any of the following signs: neck pain, numbness all over the body, nausea, light sensitivity, decreased vision, vomiting, confusion, seizures, irritability, shoulder pain, rapid loss of alertness.

A subarachnoid hemorrhage is often causally related to brain aneurysms, which are abnormalities within the brain's arteries. Other causes include use of blood thinners or a severe head injury. When an aneurysm erupts, it quickly bleeds and forms a clot. It can occur at any age, but it's most common from forty to sixty-five.

According to the Internet Stroke Center, one in fifty people in the United States is estimated to have an unruptured aneurysm. Women are more at risk than men. Some are even born with this.

A subarachnoid hemorrhage is rare, accounting for 0.08 percent of ER visits, reports the Brain Aneurysm Foundation. It is often detected during routine physicals where a doctor might note a stiff neck and vision problems. Tests include a CT scan with or without contrast, MRI, X-ray, or ultrasound. Without a scan, up to 73 percent of people are misdiagnosed.

Ischemic Stroke

An ischemic stroke occurs when arteries are blocked by blood clots or gradual buildup of plaque and fatty deposits. Stroke cuts off supplies of blood and oxygen to the brain.

Fundraisers

Introduction

When stroke took my mother's life, it found a permanent place in mine. Currently, I support stroke research and act as a source of information and prevention through my fundraisers. The events are designed to raise awareness and provide education about stroke. At the time of this publication, I have conducted three fundraisers. The proceeds support NYU Langone Medical Center's Stroke Care Center. Profits from the first fundraiser were used to publish "A Stroke Guide for Patients and Caregivers." In time, I will create more opportunities to stand in the way of this highly preventable tyrant called stroke and weaken its potential to disable and end lives.

My passion blossomed quickly; I had to start educating people about stroke. I put my love and talent for event planning to tremendous use from the start, and I continue to use those skills through each stage of executing the fundraisers. The more there is to do, the more my desire to dig in rises.

My energy soars by the day of the event; it is such an exciting process, even if it is complex and trying at times. This supposedly one-time event had me hooked. The personal fulfillment I experienced by increasing income for stroke research and education at the hospital combined with educating so many people during preparation and at the event is indescribable. All I wanted to do was step in front of a stroke and save a life, and I was doing that by a multiple that I would never know. I came to realize that my fundraiser was going to be one of many to come. My passion was so immensely aroused.

This Is for You, Mom

My beautiful mother, Eileen Bradford, passed away suddenly at the young age of sixty-two from a hemorrhagic stroke. I carry special memories of a time gone by when I lived in California with her. We were near the beach and woke every morning to go for a run along the water. I grew up in an active and health-conscious family. My mother was a physically fit and youthful woman. My life is filled with healthy choices and a wide variety of physical activities along with a focus on health coaching largely because of her positive influences. Her impressions on my life will continue to influence countless others.

I wanted to do something special for my mom and raise stroke awareness because it is so crucial to act quickly. Almost anyone can learn how to spot a stroke and then simply dial 911. To spare permanent disability or death, action must be taken immediately. I feel close to my mother when I do the fundraisers. I sense her looking down at me, sending me strength and energy to continue this mission.

I think about how my mother lost so many otherwise healthy years because stroke stopped her life so early. I will never know what may have been because nobody was there to dial 911 for her. No one was near her to simply identify her stroke symptoms and get her help.

The Birth of the Fundraisers

I called the events Fitness by the Beach. Making these events fitness-focused was a natural choice. To dovetail my passion for helping more people learn about fitness and wellness while increasing stroke awareness was an ultimate high. I was supercharged to provide these events ongoing. They encompass my greatest callings and are worthy of the effort to make them profitable for the benefactors and richly deserving for the participants. I don't know if I thought of the fundraisers or if the fundraisers came from some place bigger and just grabbed me relentlessly, knowing I was cut out for this job.

Most Saturday mornings, I took one of my favorite classes, Boot Camp by the Beach. One morning, it came to mind in a flash: *I would love to host a fitness fundraiser in memory of my mom.* I sought out hospitals with a dedicated stroke department or facility. My phone calls led me to Dr. Keith Siller at NYU Langone Medical Center's Comprehensive Stroke Care Center. We had a great conversation, and ultimately he was invested. I don't know which of us was more excited. This is an example of how things came together for me. I worked hard and certainly used my planning background, but I also received support from those I needed. I had the power to sincerely impact stroke as if I was slated to do this work all along.

Supporting Roles

Being so organized, I thought this would be easy. After all, I have produced countless corporate events, summer, and holiday parties. I had no idea how distinctive fundraisers were, they are an entirely different animal. I underestimated the extreme and diverse effort required. Fortunately, I had talent, strength, and devotion from willing friends and family, along with incredible people at the hospital.

I experienced extraordinarily high volumes in donations and raffle items. It also happened by wonderful and willing vendors and sponsors for each event. The health, fitness, and wellness vendors I approached were generous as were the healthy snack vendors who donated snacks and a water vendor who kept us hydrated with bottled water. There were numerous companies who generously contributed lovely gifts for many silent auction baskets along with other donations that we arranged by theme, such as Italian Therapy, Family Weekend, Ladies Night, Master Chef, Let's Get Physical, Night Out on the Town, and Ultimate Water Sports, just to name a few. A talented, creative close friend of mine, Rosemarie, and I created each special basket; she generously provided just what we needed from her paper and gifts business, Fleur De Lila.

More sponsors, vendors, and donations came from those I previously worked with, family, friends of friends, and even more by continuing to dial the phone and keep the e-mails going. To get the word out, I used everything at my disposal. E-mail blasts, social media like Facebook and Twitter, and I asked the participants and vendors alike to please send out an additional e-mail blast. Gary Player said, "The harder you work, the luckier you get." If you are spearheading a fundraiser, he's right.

Who, What, and Where

Orchard Beach in Rye, New York, offered a great location. Being the California native beach girl that I am, it felt right to plan the fundraisers on or overlooking a beach. From the start, I planned to tie in a physical fitness element because my mom and I were both always active.

For the second fundraiser, year two, I sought out a celebrity trainer and was lucky Joel Harper signed on. He was a crowd pleaser, and I was thrilled to have him back for season 3. I offered classes like yoga, boot camp, CrossFit, and zumba with a gorgeous ocean view and gifted each attendee with a swag bag. At the end of each event, Dr. Siller gave a talk about strokes and their causes.

I am grateful to everyone that was part of the fundraisers. I will never stop this important fight.

REAWAKENED

"Knowing others is wisdom,
knowing yourself is Enlightenment."
- Lao Tzu -

Conclusion

Change is probably the single most talked about topic on the planet, and where there is change, we find a range of emotions. We might change because our soul can't wait anymore; as Anaïs Nin said, "And the day came when the risk to remain tight in a bud was more painful than the risk it took to blossom." Other times, we have to accept change, and it becomes a matter of perspective. Franklin D. Roosevelt said, "The only thing we have to fear is fear itself." Get past the false wall of fear, and a new opportunity awaits. Don't hold yourself back and miss out on something amazing, wonderful, or perhaps a chance to change another person's life for the better. Don't allow fear to go to the grave with you.

I took you on my journey, one I never expected, one my mother seemingly set me on. I was sometimes ready to take leaps of faith, other times filled with fear. Either way, I pushed forward. Nothing served me had I stayed put. Whether you are forced into the unknown by change or considering making a change, this question can help: "What is serving me if I stay in this situation?" If you even think you might be better off by facing that fear, take a step and take it soon.

Spiritual teacher Caroline Myss explains, "The longer you wait, the greater the weight." Had I let my anxiety take over my mind, body, and life for longer, I would have remained shut in. My health and social support system would have deteriorated much more.

I will close by sharing something I truly feared. I did it to conquer it; I don't allow fear to cut experiences out of my life. It might surprise you that it wasn't a long stretch of intense schooling or a major step in my career. I was filled with fear over my ability to participate in a brutal, four-hilly mile multiple-obstacle challenge in New York called the Spartan Race. The relentless course includes repeated climbs up a mountain and recurrent scrambles up an endless hill under barbed wire, lugging heavy obstacles. It takes place annually and draws over ten thousand athletes. Spartan Races are held in multiple areas across the country.

I was working out, boxing and running, three to four times per week. I focused on my cardio early on, but the five weeks prior to the Spartan Race, I only did cardio workouts twice per week, putting time into weight training. My cardiovascular endurance was a bit weak going into this race.

For something so intense and physically testing, I knew I had not done enough training, but I went forward. In life, you never are fully prepared. You can't be. No one ever knows what's to come. You have so much more life experience than you realize, and it is amazing how it happens to be exactly what you needed for that next situation. You are made prepared for what your life hands you; let go of the word *fear*—exchange it for the word *faith*. It will get you much further.

I completed all the challenges! Beforehand, I did not understand why I had to face that fear head-on, but now I do. Once I conquered that challenge, I felt like I could do anything—a feeling that propelled me to accomplish countless greater challenges in my life. Whatever your Spartan Race may be, get ready, set, go! You are smart to not to wait! My mother inspired me to reawaken. I thank you for inspiring me to keep on helping people become their healthiest, best selves for the rest of my life.

Resources

Books

destressifying and *Secrets of Meditation* by davidji.

The Paleo Solution by Robb Wolf, thepaleodiet.com

Integrative Nutrition by Joshua Rosenthal

Superfoods, the Food and Medicine of the Future by David Wolfe

Mind Your Body: 4 Weeks to a Leaner, Healthier Life by Joel Harper

The Secret by Rhonda Byrne

10% Happier by Dan Harris

The Immune System Recovery Plan by Susan Blum and Mark Hyman

The Wheel of Healing with Ayurveda by Michelle S. Fondin

Healing Spices by Bharat B. Aggarwal, PhD, Debora Yost

Meditation

To get a sense of mindfulness meditation, try one of Dr. Ronald Siegel's guided recordings. They are available at no charge at www.mindfulness-solution.com. Davidji offers guided meditations and a host of meditation information at davidji.com.

DVD

Qigong for Beginners by Chris Pei.

Panic and Anxiety Disorder

National Panic and Anxiety Disorder News.com

Bibliography

Carbonell Phd, David. "Beat the Anxiety Trick: How to Overcome Chronic Anxiety." Anxietycoach.com, 10 Mar. 2016. Web. 25 Mar. 2016.

Bardot, JB. "25 Powerful Reasons to Eat Bananas." *Food Matters*, 14 Aug. 2012. Web. 13 Apr. 2016.

Desta, Yohana. "10 Famous Writers Who Don't Use Modern Tech to Create." Mashable, 15 Feb. 2014. Web. 1 Apr. 2016.

Desta, Yohana. "7 Ways Writing by Hand Can save Your Brain." Mashable, 19 Jan. 2015. Web. 14 Feb. 2016.

Maria Konnikova, "What's Lost as Handwriting Fades," p. D1. *The New York Times*, New York ed., June 3, 2014.

Anne Chemin, "Handwriting vs typing: is the pen still mightier than the keyboard?" *The Guardian*, December 16, 2014.

Kissel Wegela Phd, Karen. "How to Practice Mindfulness Meditation." *Psychology Today*. 19 Jan. 2010. Web. 3 Feb. 2016.

"What Is Qigong?" National Qigong Association, n.d. Web. 13 Mar. 2016.

Cohen, Kenneth. "Benefits of Self-Healing Qigong." Sacred Earth Circle, 2009. Web. 16 Apr. 2016.

Health Coaching. *World Class Health Coaching*. Institute for Integrative Nutrition, n.d. Web. 20 Apr. 2016.

Jonathan Wright, Linda Johnson Larsen, *Eating Clean for Dummies*, 2nd ed., August 2016.

"Vinyasa." Learn About Vinyasa Yoga: Poses, Asanas & Sequences. *Yoga Journal*, n.d. Web. 5 Jan. 2016.

Haines, Jenna. "10 Professional Athletes Who Practice Yoga." Men's Fitness, n.d. Web. 23 Feb. 2016.

Zirm, Jordan. "10 Athletes and Teams You Might Not Think Would Practice Yoga." *Stack*, 17 Sept. 2012. Web. 23 Feb. 2016.

Richard Rosen, "Here Comes the Sun: The Tradition of Surya Namaskar." *Yoga Journal*, August 28, 2007.

"Ayurveda." Central Council of Indian Medicine, n.d. Web. 26 Feb. 2016.

"Bachelor of Ayurvedic Medicine and Surgery (BAMS)." Career in BAMS: How to Become an Ayurvedic Doctor? *Sarvgyan*, n.d. Web. 4 Apr. 2016.

"Ayurveda—The Science of Life."*Ayurveda | The Chopra Center*. n.p., n.d. Web. 3 Mar. 2016.

"Stroke Facts." National Stroke Association, n.d. Web. 10 Mar. 2016. Stroke.org.

"What is Stroke?" National Stroke Association, n.d. Web. 10 Mar. 2016. *Stroke.org*.

Notes

CPSIA information can be obtained
at www.ICGtesting.com
Printed in the USA
BVOW05s1630300317

479879BV00013B/71/P